# STARCH MADNESS

"What to eat . . . and why . . . a book well worth reading if you wish to take charge of your health."
    Barry Sears, Ph.D.
    author, *The Zone* and *Mastering the Zone*

"I have enjoyed reading *Starch Madness* and find it helpful in managing my own eating habits. Your thesis certainly makes a lot of sense. I am sure that my father would have approved of your ideas also, just as he did back in 1987. I think your book will prove itself to be a great source of information for those who are concerned with diet and well-being."
    Linus Pauling, Jr., M.D.

"Not a 'quick fix' diet book, but a lifelong program for optimal nutrition and natural weight loss. Mr. Heinrich explains why most popular diets don't work—and what does."
    Julian Whitaker, M.D.
    editor, *Health & Healing*

"*Starch Madness* is truly a superior health diet book we should all read more than once. It is an in-depth rendition of the ultimate truth on diet and perfect health."
    Fereydoon Batmanghelidj, M.D.
    author, *Your Body's Many Cries for Water*

"*Starch Madness* gives a useful and balanced assessment of many of the diets which have been suggested, not just to improve weight loss, but to lead to general good health. Are you confused about what you should eat? Richard Heinrich provides a guide which just about any reader can benefit from. His book is on my recommended reading list."
    Dallas Clouatre, Ph.D.
    author, *Getting Lean with Anti-fat Nutrients*

***Starch Madness* is a modern eating primer** . . . taken straight from the eating patterns of our Paleolithic ancestors, who ate the foods supplied directly by Mother Nature.

This book, *Starch Madness,* provides scientific state-of-the-art facts that relate to all foods. It thoroughly documents **human eating patterns that date back to Paleolithic times** and is a well-reasoned, daily guide on **how to eat.**

**"Starch Madness" has created the fattest society in world history,** the pasta-mad United States of America. We eat too much, our foods are loaded with calories, we have too much stress, and we don't exercise. *No wonder we don't "feel good!"*

**We must learn who and what we are.** First, stand back to contemplate evolution. *Our genes are from the stone age.* For eons, man ate a low-glycemic, protein-rich diet. Now we eat diets loaded with sugar, refined starches, and saturated fat.

**It is pure "starch madness" to eat five times more starch than protein,** as recommended by current interpretations of pyramid-type diets. This guarantees high insulin levels—the number one predictor of heart problems—which prevent fat cells from releasing fat, and lower blood sugar levels, thus creating more fat. When hungry, you will eat still more starch to keep up the "starch madness" rhythm.

**Learn the correct ratio to balance blood sugar *and* access body fat for energy.** Eating three to five times more carbohydrate than protein means "fat" (flabby fat with lack of muscle fiber). When you eat correctly, you won't know you're hungry, because you are living off all that body fat. **Learn *why* and *how* this happens.**

Excess insulin caused by **"starch madness"** can be dangerous to your health. **The proper carbohydrate-protein ratio** can eliminate the need for drugs, medicines, and petty addictions for caffeine and candy—even smoking!

**The author's blood profile is reported on page 61.** Now (Sept. 16, 1998) his HDL cholesterol is 74, reported by the Cooper Clinic, up from 67 last year and 54 before the Zone diet. No drugs, just protein/carbohydrate, fat balance.

*Starch Madness* explains and resolves the differences between the pyramid-type high starch diets, the sugar deluge diets, the low fat diets, and the controlled protein diets. The Zone is proven the winner in background and concept. . . .

**Learn how much fat** of which type is vital. This book preaches low fat, and "good" and "bad" fats—and how to remain well within American Heart Association guidelines.

**Learn why water** is a main ingredient in our health program, and how lack of water can cause disease and even addictions.

**Learn why the diseases of civilization**—blocked blood vessels, high blood pressure, asthma, joint pain, cancer, dental problems etc.—are all caused by an imbalanced diet and a chronic lack of water.

**Learn how to eat** the diet that has fed and nourished humankind for 99 percent of our existence.

**Learn to empower yourself** with proper diet, and reap the many rewards—a longer life, a happier disposition, freedom from depression and compelling addictions, greater physical agility and youthfulness, and a clear mind. *Eating the right foods is the secret.*

**Learn the teachings** of the most renowned experts on health, wellness, and diet of the last 50 years. All their knowledge is summarized and synthesized in *Starch Madness*. You can become (again) a healthy, whole person, vital and energetic.

**Learn how to take intelligent control** of the health and well-being of your own body.

**Turn to Chapter 12** for "MY DIET PRIMER."

**Turn to page 106** and following for DIET TIPS and a Lifetime Maintenance Diet.

**Turn to page 133** for GUIDELINES FOR WEIGHT CONTROL

*from Starch Madness:*

"This book pays rightful homage to the 'wellness prophets' of the twentieth century who perceived ahead of their time the link between our diet and our daily-life health."

"If Barry Sears' *Zone* is the new diet testament, then the words of Adelle Davis are the old testament, and Linus Pauling the prophet. If Dr. Kenneth Cooper's aerobics and his whole wellness series are the new wellness testament, then Dr. Hans Selye's work on stress is the old testament and Dr. George Sheehan the prophet."

"This is not nostalgia for the good old days, nor is it a plea for natural foods, and certainly not for vegetarianism, all of which seem to lead to—grain. It is a plea to consider the 'facts' that modern science has taught us about early mankind . . . and how our genetic constitution has evolved from biological processes eons earlier."

"When you complete your own 'diet primer'—as detailed in this book—you will see that starch foods can be eaten, but in limited amounts that do not curtail your intake of fibers, vitamins, and minerals."

"The mealtime conviviality of dining with family and friends, even the gustatory sensations when eating alone, are partially dependent on the time spent eating and the amount of chewing. Ergo, learn to eat the almost unlimited amount of low glycemic foods, thus keeping you laughing and sparkling at parties, instead of fattening up from overeating starches."

"I have found two venues for wellness: the *Zone Diet* and *exercise*. The Zone diet will consume your fat, albeit a bit slower, without exercise. But the two are so inseparable that, if you can develop the discipline to accomplish one, you *can* accomplish the other."

"*Can you afford to wait?* The goal for all of us, at whatever age, is to achieve and enjoy a lifestyle that will enhance our life today . . . and tomorrow."

# STARCH MADNESS

## Paleolithic Nutrition for Today

*with a Foreword by*
Barry Sears, Ph.D.
author of *The Zone* and *Mastering the Zone*

### Richard L. Heinrich

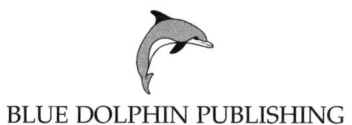

BLUE DOLPHIN PUBLISHING

*Disclaimer*: This book is not intended to replace medical advice or the care of a physician. The author and publisher expressly disclaim responsibility for any adverse effects arising from dietary procedures which this book discusses. If you are taking a prescription medication, do not change your diet without first consulting your physician.

When launching a diet or exercising for fitness, medical advice is a must. While the author provides personal anecdotes that correlate to research quoted in this book, the reader must make a personal and informed decision.

Copyright 1999 © Richard L. Heinrich
All rights reserved.

Published by Blue Dolphin Publishing, Inc.
P.O. Box 8, Nevada City, CA 95959
Orders: 1-800-643-0765

ISBN: 1-57733-027-7

Library of Congress Cataloging-in-Publication Data

Heinrich, Richard L.
    starch madness : paleolithic nutrition for today / Richard L. Heinrich : with a foreword by Barry Sears
      p.    cm.
    Includes bibliographical references and index.
    ISBN 1-57733-027-7 (alk. paper)
    1. Reducing diets.    I. Title.
RM222.2.H343  1999
613.2'5—dc21                                    98-33637
                                                                 CIP

Cover photo: Author chomping tomato
                by granddaughter, Jennifer Ann Neck

Cover design: Lito Castro

Printed in the United States of America

10   9   8   7   6   5   4   3   2   1

*Dedicated to*
*Mary Wells Bardwell*
*Steamboat Springs, Colorado*

Without *The Zone* book gift from Mary, *this book* would never have seen print. Our karma carries back 54 years, even before the trailer housing at Camp Randall in Madison that knew Ann and Becky and Roger. Mary, we love you and now publicly avow it.

Richard L. Heinrich
Delafield, Wisconsin
March 31, 1998

*Paleolithic:* Early Stone Age, beginning approximately 750,000 years ago and ending 15,000 years ago.

*Editor's Note:* Congratulations for picking up *Starch Madness* and learning why and how we should eat to live a long, healthy life. To achieve the greatest satisfaction in reading this book, start with the Glossary, then glance at the Bibliography, then contemplate the Reading List. This book gives you a grounding in all of the Reading List teachings.

Now glance at the Contents and Illustrations, read the Foreword, Preface and Wind Up. Finally, all the chapters stand by themselves, and there is a flow, but try to read a complete chapter at a sitting.

# CONTENTS

| | | |
|---|---|---|
| List of Illustrations | | x |
| Foreword | | xiii |
| Preface | | xv |
| Chapter 1 | The Evolutionary Diet | 1 |
| Chapter 2 | The Low Fat Diet | 11 |
| Chapter 3 | The Low Glycemic Diet | 18 |
| Chapter 4 | The Training Table | 34 |
| Chapter 5 | Barry Sears: The Zone | 49 |
| Chapter 6 | The Promised Land | 66 |
| Chapter 7 | Your Body's Many Cries for Water | 72 |
| Chapter 8 | The New Nutrition | 76 |
| Chapter 9 | Taking Stress in Stride | 82 |
| Chapter 10 | And the Word Was Aerobics | 87 |
| Chapter 11 | Fitness – Fatness – Wellness | 91 |
| Chapter 12 | My Diet Primer | 97 |
| Chapter 13 | A Call to Arms | 109 |
| Chapter 14 | The Windup | 113 |
| Appendix 1 | Fat-Cholesterol List | 123 |
| Appendix 2 | Optimal Nutrition | 125 |
| Appendix 3 | Suggested Reading List | 135 |
| Glossary | | 137 |
| Bibliography | | 140 |
| Index | | 143 |

# ILLUSTRATIONS

| | | |
|---|---|---|
| Table 1 | Comparison of the Late Paleolithic Diet, the Current American Diet, and U.S. Dietary Recommendations | 6 |
| Table 2 | Absolute Daily Amounts of the Macronutrients in Grams | 8 |
| Fig. 1 | Curves Demonstrating Response to Glucose Leading to Glycemic Index Ratings | 21 |
| Fig. 2 | Curves Showing Response to Glucose of Obese vs. Thin Subjects | 24 |
| Fig. 3 | Curves Showing Response to Glucose of a Maturity Onset Diabetic | 25 |
| Fig. 4 | Male and Female Death Rates in Various Countries for Coronary Heart Disease | 26 |
| Table 3 | Glycemic Index for Different Carbohydrates | 27 |
| Table 4 | Classification of Carbohydrates | 28 |
| Table 5 | Classification of Foods as Macronutrients | 29 |
| Table 6 | Classification of Allowed Foods for Montignac Weight Loss Diet | 30 |
| Table 7 | Classification of Allowed Foods for Montignac Weight Maintenance Diet | 31 |

| | | |
|---|---|---|
| Table 8 | Recommended Protein and Fat Grams for Various Diets | 54 |
| Table 9 | Comparison of Zone Reducing Diet and Real Life Diet | 55 |
| Fig. 5 | Pictorial Portrayal of the Zone | 56 |
| Table 10 | Protein and Fat Gram Typical Sources from Netzer Food Counts | 100 |
| Table 11 | Macronutrient Gram Make-up for Typical Fast Foods from Netzer Food Counts | 101 |

.

# FOREWORD

What should you eat? Americans have never been more confused. One study will contradict the latest "breakthrough" published only weeks earlier. The government says fat is the villain, and Americans are eating less fat now than at any time in recent history. Yet we have become the fattest people on the face of the earth. How is it possible? Is there no rhyme or reason in the nutrition universe?

Richard Heinrich has stepped into this void and has pulled together an excellent survey of new approaches to this seemingly age-old problem of what to eat, and more importantly, why. It all starts with our genes that haven't changed in the last 100,000 years and are unlikely to change in the near future. The correct diet for Americans (and all humans for that matter) is based on what is genetically correct, not politically correct.

I am very appreciative that my research on the Zone Diet has been included in this work. For once you can understand the genetic boundaries for a hormonally correct diet—you can now develop food as an exceptionally powerful drug—a 21st-century drug to control hormonal responses that are hundreds of times more powerful than any pharmaceutical known.

With such knowledge we can finally understand what Hippocrates, the father of medicine, meant 2,500 years ago when he stated, "Let food be your medicine; let medicine be your food." As we enter into a new millennium, food has the power to alter our health care system completely. However, the door can swing both ways. If we continue to ignore our genetic make-up and the hormonal consequences of the diet, our existing health care may end up in shambles within a few decades. *Starch Madness* is a book well worth reading and studying if you wish to empower yourself to take charge of your destiny.

—Barry Sears, Ph.D.

# PREFACE

I am seventy-two. I have always had a weight problem. Withal I stayed in bounds, but with a struggle, trying out every diet pattern, while observing my slender friends seemingly pack in more food than any calorie-counting eating pattern should allow. I am sure that this is a common observation for those of us afflicted with what I now recognize as Paleolithic genes.

Four years ago I learned of a diet book by Michel Montignac, a business executive whose *Dine Out and Lose Weight* has been a best seller in France since 1987. Critics were calling this just another high protein regimen. *But I was transfixed by my first exposure to the glycemic index.*

Of course I knew about simple sugars and complex carbohydrates and the current popularity of pasta, pasta, pasta. Ye gods, even pasta salad, a misnomer if ever I heard of one. But suddenly pasta, potatoes, and refined starches were equated with simple sugar in that they all caused equal production of insulin, creating fat, lowering blood sugar, creating hunger, and keeping the cycle going.

Now I have been through very successful protein/fat diets but always gained the unwanted pounds after getting back to "normalcy" eating pasta, pasta, pasta. Montignac offers a life's eating pattern that is keeping me within bounds: low glycemic carbohydrates with protein/lipids. What is the proof of this? Is it good for you?

Just at this time I read *The Paleolithic Prescription* by S.B. Eaton, M. Shostak and M. Konner. The light dawned. This low-glycemic diet is the diet of our ancestors, of prehistory, learned through the millennia. It is the diet that mankind evolved eating. What has messed up mankind is pasta, pasta, pasta. And sugar, sugar, sugar. Each equates to the other.

My most recent diet was fat-gram restricting. I reviewed Martin Katahn's book, *T-Factor Diet*, admired it, and certainly suggest it as required reading. However, for me, after being told to *Eat, eat carbohydrates,* and going around with a nose bag of pretzels all day, it didn't work—I was always hungry. I think there are many people for whom it won't work. To eat complex carbohydrates like pasta, pasta, pasta has proven to be as bad as sugar, sugar, sugar and is a sure way to obesity for most of us.

I wrote to the *Runner's World Forum* in 1976 on the subject of macronutrient mix and insulin production, ending with *"the whole situation screams for decent research,"* and again in 1994 to the Cooper Clinic, ending with *"hopefully diets will be tailored to insulin production."* **That new era has arrived with Barry Sears, Ph.D., and** *The Zone, A Dietary Road Map.* He has explained the complex biochemistry of nutrition and demonstrated the proportions of nutrients needed to produce the hormonal reactions of well being. I believe he has conquered the diseases of civilization, of course making use of much research of others, but recognizing the elegant unity of disease to nutrition. And, his "diet" brought me down to the weight I was at 17.

This new diet information resolved for me the wellness dilemma and convinced me that I should expand the testaments that I had already written for my sons on my "heroes of fitness"—my books to live by.

If Barry Sears' Zone is the new diet testament, then the words of Adelle Davis are the old testament, and Linus Pauling the prophet. If Dr. Kenneth Cooper's aerobics and his whole wellness series are the new wellness testament, then Dr. Hans Selye's work on stress is the old testament and Dr. George Sheehan the prophet.

Adelle Davis was arguably the nation's best known nutritionist in the 1950-60s. Today her books are very much in print as Penguin paperbacks. I had written a synopsis of her *Let's Eat Right to Keep Fit* circa 1964, and in reviewing this after learning about Barry Sears' Zone, noted how serendipitous are its precepts. The genius of Barry Sears set the proportions of carbohydrate/protein/fat that create a life's eating regimen that will produce slenderness. Sears is a pioneer in biotechnology (12 patents) who has presented the world with "The Zone," described in Chapter Five.

Nobel prize winner Linus Pauling, Ph.D., capped his seventy-year active career with studies of micronutrients described in Chapter Seven. Again, the serendipity of the Zone diet produces the orthomolecular medicine of wellness on which Linus Pauling spent his last years.

Dr. Kenneth Cooper's aerobics were my salvation. Chapter Nine defines "the conditioned person," the work of Dr. Cooper, who, as a colonel in the Air Force, surmised his insights into fitness and proved them for humanity in 1968. He quantified fitness, showing how aerobic points translate directly into the pulse rate and blood pressure of true health. I joined in as I do to this day—best Cooper Clinic treadmill time, 23.10 min. at age 59. I commenced my lifetime subscription to *Runner's World* magazine and was introduced to cardiologist and runner Dr. George Sheehan. His several books make him the guru, the philosopher of fitness.

From Dr. Sheehan, I learned of the work of Dr. Hans Selye, whose biography and work are described in Chapter Eight. And I understand *why* fitness equates to mental health, both the body *and* the mind. And I read Dr. Sheehan's list of *his* books to live by: the philosopher Ortega Y. Gasset, but also *The Paleolithic Prescription* of scholars Eaton, Shostak, and Konner described in Chapter One. And I have come full circle.

I *believe* that I have arrived at a basic diet *truth*. I *believe* that I have arrived at a basic mental health *truth*. I *believe* that I have provided a clarity of analysis and presentation in this book that will coordinate the sometimes disparate writings of the great minds of my era into a unity—a unity that all can understand.

I present my health-heroes of the past half-century, and their thoughts, to awaken your own mental and physical well-being.

# STARCH MADNESS

Paleolithic Nutrition for Today

# 1

# THE EVOLUTIONARY DIET

**The Paleolithic Prescription**
S. Boyd Eaton, M.D., Marjorie Shostak &
Melvin Konner, M.D., Ph.D. (HarperCollins, 1988)
**The Driving Force, Food, Evolution, and the Future**
M. Crawford & David Marsh (HarperCollins, 1989)
**"Paleolithic Nutrition: A Consideration of
Its Nature and Current Implications"**
S. Boyd Eaton & Melvin Konner
*(New England Journal of Medicine, 1985, 312: 283-289)*

Our evolution over the eons has provided us with a digestive system which is based upon foods of the Paleolithic era and earlier. We can term our very genes Paleolithic, evolved to flourish from hunter-gatherer eating patterns. Only about 25% of humankind has adapted a body able to cope with the foods of the Age of Agriculture without obesity and all of its problems. "The diet of our remote ancestors may be a reference standard for modern human nutrition and a model for defense against certain *diseases of civilization!*" (Eaton & Konner, 1985, p. 288).

We discuss the diseases of civilization at three locations in this book. In this chapter, to give a definition and background, in Chapter Five to explain how the Zone diet can help resolve them, and in Chapter Seven to show how insufficient water exacerbates them. These factors, plus weight control, may well put you on the road to renewed health. Here are the maladies wrought by the lifestyle and diet of modern man, diseases that are perpetually treated but, all too often, not cured:

- Atherosclerosis, blood vessel blockage underlying most strokes and heart attacks
- Hypertension, high blood pressure
- Obesity and adult onset diabetes
- Chronic lung disease
- Cancer
- Alcohol related disease
- Smoking
- Dental caries
- Diverticulitis

*The different diseases set against different nutritional backgrounds of the different countries tell us first, that nutrition has a profound effect on human physiology and performance. Secondly, they tell us that the change in food composition has occurred at a rate too fast for any selective response. . . . The response to the rapid change in food structure is being expressed in the form of atherosclerosis* (Crawford & Marsh, 1989, p. 246).

We know, we all know, that self-control of our daily living will assist in reversing this litany of debilitation. Let us try to reason how our modern diet and addictions differ from our ancestors.

Our diet, derived from the age of agriculture, covers only the last 10,000 years. And the age of agriculture is the age of high caloric density starch plants. It is biblical, with bread the staff of life. The very meaning of the word "ingrained" (even if its etymology comes from wood grain) tells us how firmly fixed is the belief that grain stands supreme (7 to 11 daily servings in the Food Pyramid Diet).

Grain permitted a great population expansion, which, with a lack of animal foods, caused short stature due to poor nutrition. Man lost about 6 inches of height. Only today are we back to the 5'10" males and 5'6" females of the Stone Age. Grain brought animal husbandry to smaller population areas, allowing better nutrition. But with the dairy products came domesticated meats with vastly greater fat content. And then came sugar, and now the ersatz foods and combinations designed for packaging and long shelf-life.

This is not nostalgia for the good old days, nor is it a plea for natural foods, and certainly not for vegetarianism, all of which seem to lead to—grain. It is a plea to consider the facts that modern science has taught us about early mankind. Let us now look back in time.

Our genetic constitution has changed little in 10,000 years; its make-up evolved from biological processes eons earlier. "Evolution has conserved this system (insulin, glucagon, and the eicosanoids) for hundreds of millions of years, and made it standard operating equipment for an amazingly wide variety of species, including man" (Sears, 1995, p. 100). Proto-humans evolved about 5 million years ago, began using stone tools 2 million years ago, and ate meat. The staggering flow of time is apparent when we consider generations:

- Computers       -   1 generation
- Industrial      -   10 generations
- Agriculture     -   500 generations
- Homo sapiens    -   20,000 generations
- Hunter gatherers -  100,000 generations

Ninety-nine percent of our genetic heritage dates back to before the appearance of humankind. Only one percent of our biological makeup has appeared since human and great ape lines separated some seven million years ago. The point is to reflect upon how little has been the opportunity to adapt our body to the age of agriculture.

*Looking at the scene of human nutrition from this perspective it is obvious that throughout human evolution, man relied on wild foods. His physiology was initially adapted by, and is still adapted to, wild not modern foods. He spent 99.8 percent of his existence as a species living on wild foods* (Crawford & Marsh, 1989, p. 257).

Paleo-anthropologists have surmised bodily make-up and diets from skeletal remains, and game bone remains. Modern hunter-gatherers have been studied. From this we learn that pre-agricultural people were robust and about today's size. Their lives were short, perhaps 18 years on average. Even in Roman times, the average age was about 22, but we know that some people lived to be very old. The population at 8,000 BC, about the beginning of agriculture, was 8 million. By 1,500 AD, it had become 350 million, and now will soon exceed 7 billion.

Table 1 shows the diet that our bodies evolved to follow and compares it to the 1985 American diet. It is revealing indeed. Amounts shown are percentages. The foods we eat and the physical exercise we engage in have changed radically, particularly since the industrial revolution. The Paleolithic diet is estimated to be 35% meat and

65% plant food. The meat was lean with little saturated fat, but contained the same levels of cholesterol as today, since cholesterol is found largely in cell membranes. Examine the late Paleolithic diet in comparison to the two modern diets:

- Protein consumption was 3 times higher, carbohydrate was about the same, and fat was much lower, about 50% of today's diet.
- The ratio of carbohydrate to protein was 4 to 3, exactly as recommended by Barry Sears in the Zone Diet, but much lower than that recommended by the *Consumer Reports* 1992 diet, which is more than 6 to 1.
- Fat intake was lower than today's diet, actually equal in grams to the 1992 *Consumer Reports* consensus diet.
- P/S Ratio (polyunsaturated fat to saturated fat) was about the ideal recommended today. The reason for this was (and is) that wild game meat had much less fat and the fat was less saturated. Eaton and Konner point out that fat from the cape buffalo is about equally split between saturated, unsaturated, and polyunsaturated, and "assume a similar ratio for wild game in general" (Eaton & Konner, 1985, p. 286). Keep this in mind as you read on. It is another powerful reason to emulate the Paleolithic diet. Today protein food selections should be made from foods that maximize unsaturated fat. See Appendix One.
- Cholesterol was equal to today, but double that recommended today. Cholesterol is found in connective tissue, not in fat.
- Fiber intake was much higher. Today's standard diet will not yield today's recommended amount.

- Calcium intake was much higher even without dairy foods.
- Vitamin C at an estimated 400 milligrams was about seven times greater than the recommended amount a few years ago.
- Potassium ingestion was much higher and sodium much lower, as potassium is leached out in modern food preparation. Salt is now added constantly.
- Total energy was 34% protein, 21% fat, and 45% carbohydrate.
- There were no refined grains, milk, or sugar.

### TABLE 1
### Comparison of the Late Paleolithic Diet,* the Current American Diet, and U.S. Dietary Recommendations

| | LATE PALEOLITHIC DIET* | U.S. SENATE CURRENT AMERICAN DIET | SELECT COMMITTEE RECOMMENDATIONS |
|---|---|---|---|
| Total dietary energy (%) | | | |
| Protein | 34 | 12 | 12 |
| Carbohydrate | 45 | 46 | 58 |
| Fat | 21 | 42 | 30 |
| P:S ratio † | 1.41 | 0.44 | 1.00 |
| Cholesterol (mg) | 591 | 600 | 300 |
| Fiber (g) | 45.7 | 19.7 ‡ | 30-60 |
| Sodium (mg) | 690 | 2300-6900 | 1100-3300 |
| Calcium (mg) | 1580 | 740 § | 800-1200 ¶ |
| Ascorbic acid (mg) | 392.3 | 87.7 § | 45 ¶ |

\* Assuming the diet contained 35 per cent meat and 65 per cent vegetables.
† P:S denotes polyunsaturated: saturated fats.
‡ British National Food Survey, 1976.
§ U.S. Department of Agriculture Food Consumption Survey, 1977-1978.
¶ Recommended Daily Dietary Allowance, Food and Nutrition Board, National Academy of Sciences-National Research Council.

Reprinted by permission from "Paleolithic Nutrition," Eaton & Konner, Jan. 31, 1985, *New England Journal of Medicine and Surgery*.

Copyright, 1985, Massachusetts Medical Society, All Rights Reserved.

Paleontologists studying ancient campsites have determined that there were times of plenty and times of scarcity. Today's hunter-gatherers give us a possible pattern of Stone Age eating and work practices. We have been programmed through the eons to overeat in times of plenty. It is entirely sensible to fatten up for the lean times, and those of us with this ability could survive the best. *We obese are survivors!*, so to say. We must create lean times by reducing intake and by learning a pattern of eating that will provide stability.

Today's hunter-gatherers do not gain weight and lose muscle tone as they age. The activity pattern of work days/rest days creates both endurance and strength. Fitness provides diet control, fat loss, and muscle gain, and helps retain body composition through a lifetime. Although many diet books dismiss exercise as a means of weight loss, it is a fact that 100 calories consumed by exercise each day will add up to ten pounds of fat loss in a year. Body composition and muscularity are of greater consequence than mere weight loss. It is important to lose fat and gain muscle. Men should strive for 15% body fat, women, 25%. Body strength exercise increases bone density, reducing the likelihood of osteoporosis. It also reduces the likelihood of backache.

We must learn what we are. Our genes are of the Stone Age, but we try to remain healthy in a twentieth century that has brought a life of softness and plenty. We eat too much; we don't exercise. We eat too much salt and too little calcium. We overload on sugar and forget fiber. We eat "pasta, pasta, pasta," and forget green vegetables. We ingest too little vitamin C and vitamin B and should take a supplement. Our foods are loaded with calories. We overeat before we know we are full. We eat more fat but surprisingly about the same amount of cholesterol. We eat much less protein but are told it's still too much. We are told that it is natural to gain weight and lose fitness and muscle as we get old. And not very old!

Can we get back to basics? I believe that defining the basics is a big first step and that my lifetime's heroes can teach us new patterns of diet and health.

It is instructive to compare absolute amounts of the macronutrients—protein, fat, and carbohydrates—in the Stone Age to today. Even with wide variation in total calories, the absolute amounts can give us insights into their health.

Table 2 compares six diets. The Paleolithic Diet, the 1985 American Diet, and Senate Recommended Diet are from Table 1 and are averages. The Cooper Clinic Real Life Diet is explained in Chapter Five. The *Consumer Reports* 1992 Diet is a consensus of nutrition experts, for which a ratio of nutrients is inferred to be 25% fat, 12% protein, and 63% carbohydrate *(Consumer Reports,* Oct. 1992, p. 644-651). The Sears Zone Reducing Diet, shown for comparison, has proportions figured for the proverbial average man since the other Table 2 diets are also averages.

### TABLE 2
### Absolute Daily Amounts of the Macronutrients in Grams

| | CALORIES | PROTEIN | FAT | CARBOHYDRATE |
|---|---|---|---|---|
| Paleolithic | 3000 | 255 | 70 | 337 |
| Cooper Real Life | 2500 | 116 | 107 | 268 |
| Current American | 2500 | 75 | 117 | 287 |
| Senate Recommended | 2500 | 75 | 83 | 362 |
| 1992 *Consumer Reports* | 2500 | 75 | 69 | 394 |
| Sears Zone (154 lb. average man, moderately active) Reducing Diet | 1002 | 77 | 33 | 99 |

The Paleolithic diet was determined to be 3000 calories, which, using the historic figure of 15 calories per pound of body weight, would be the proper amount for my 200 pounds. However, a more realistic figure today would be 2500 calories. Thus the other eating patterns are based on 2500, with nutrient amounts factored from the percent ratios given for each diet. The reader can adjust the amounts based on his or her weight.

These rather laborious figures are presented at this time to develop the broad themes of this book. Current media practice is to extol carbohydrates and denigrate both fat and protein. Now, Table 2 shows that for eons protein was far, far higher than today and that the consensus amount of protein in modern diets equals that for the proverbial average man, moderately active, in the Zone Diet. Later, you will learn how to figure your own protein requirement. This vital daily need is identical for both a reducing or life's eating regimen. A reducing diet that cuts half the calories and also half the protein will reduce this vital nutrient such that your own muscle tissue is consumed.

Fat grams in the Paleolithic era diet were lower than today, and these were predominantly good fat. You will learn about "good" and "bad" fat, and that fat is a vital daily need, not to be cut without careful study.

Carbohydrate intake was close to today's recommended amounts. You will learn a great deal about carbohydrate. It is important to examine a carbohydrate's makeup, its glycemic "density," and whether it has vitamins, minerals, fibers. Paleolithic man ate 3 to 5 pounds of vegetables and fruits daily! They got to 337 grams the hard way. We, on the other hand, eat "pasta, pasta, pasta."

You will also learn what nutrients to keep and which to discard.

Simply reducing calories must reduce weight, but more slowly than is logical. Katahn (1989, p. 25) tells us that in its conservation mode, metabolic processes are slow or sluggish. We withstand these diets, but we don't feel well and revert to our "standard" diet when we have lost our target weight.

For not quite a lifetime, I have had the frustration of gaining back the pounds lost on a successful diet. Now I have presented the perhaps comforting concept of our Paleolithic genes. We will learn in Chapter Three how the glycemic index of carbohydrates leads two-thirds of us into the yo-yo diet syndrome. Diets work, but then they fail.

*Chapter Five will teach us how the Zone diet provides a ratio of macro nutrients to permit at long last eating sharply reduced calories successfully—without hunger. The resulting glucagon/ insulin ratio actually promotes burning of body fat, which use is much curtailed in high starch ratio diets because of high insulin.*

We will see in Chapter Eleven that fatness with fitness may be acceptably healthy, but can we put this knowledge of evolutionary diet to use in creating leanness and wellness? of creating mental equanimity?

Yes, we can. Let us initially consider in Chapter Two the diet that works for the third of us who have adapted to the age of agriculture.

# 2

# THE LOW FAT DIET

*T-Factor Diet,* Martin Katahn (W.W. Norton & Co., 1989)
*Let's Eat Right to Keep Fit,* Adelle Davis
(Harcourt-Brace & Co., 1954)

It is amazing to read Adelle Davis again; it was all there in 1954, all the sensible stuff on cholesterol, sugar, insulin, and diet. Her amazing prescience on the roles of the macronutrients, the importance of their mix on cholesterol and insulin, starches equating to sugar—all were seemingly lost to the mainstream myopic view of fat and cholesterol (a provocative statement, but read on: Barry Sears' Zone is actually lower than the Pyramid diet in cholesterol and fat).

Considering the guff of the past forty years, what are we to believe? It appears that each proponent of a diet theory simply tries to proselytize. Each new "study" is given sensational publicity. Nutritionists become overnight experts after chalking up a few three-credit courses.

After years of recommended daily allowances and balanced diets, the establishment now recommends antioxidants and the ubiquitous "Food Pyramid." As the arguments over cholesterol and sugar are not much different than in Adelle Davis' day, what conclusions can we draw?

Let us examine three diets for weight loss and maintenance: Katahn's Low Fat diet, Montignac's Low Glycemic diet, and the Zone by Barry Sears. We build to the Zone in the sequence that I learned about it. The thrusts of these diets are in opposition, but there are points of similarity and value in each. Their facts are properly presented and each may function for you—your body "shape" may decide. We will learn that, for most of us, calorie counting diets (the high-starch, pyramid-type diets) are doomed to failure because our blood sugar is not stabilized. The resultant over-production of insulin prevents the use of body fat and creates hunger even with a plethora of starch calories.

Katahn's diet is a low fat/unlimited carbohydrate approach; Montignac's is a low glycemic diet with relatively higher protein/lipid. **And finally, the Zone by Sears resolves the conflicts between Adelle Davis' day and the new century, and truly offers a new method for living in the wellness zone.**

Each diet "works" within certain parameters. This book's thesis is to define these parameters and compare and relate them to the eating patterns of our genetic heritage.

According to Martin Katahn (1989):
- Only fat makes you fat.
- Hunger results from lack of carbohydrates.
- Don't be hungry.
- Eat as much of nonfat foods whenever you want.

- Calories don't count so don't count calories.
- Count fat grams until you have settled on a low fat diet and know the procedure. When dieting, limit fat grams to about 20 to 30 per day for women and 30 to 40 for men. When maintaining your Thin-factor (T-Factor) body, increase limit to 40 grams for women, 60 for men. These fat grams are about half of what the average person now eats.

The three metabolic factors are:
- Thermic effects of foods. A whopping 97 percent of carbohydrate is consumed in digestion, only 3 percent of fat and 25 percent of protein. (Within the normal range of our diet, says Katahn, protein is not a weight factor as it will be used in our daily fuel mixture).
- Thermic effect of exercise. Aerobics directly burn fat and indirectly increase metabolism.
- Adaptive thermogenesis. The body conserves, and it wastes. In its conserving mode, metabolic processes are slowed. In its wasteful mode, eating plentiful carbohydrates increases the metabolism and keeps you in overdrive.

Annotated from *T-Factor Diet* (Katahn, 1989, pp. 24-41) by permission of W.W. Norton, Co.

The body stores about 2000 calories in glycogen (carbohydrate), turning half of this over each day. The glycogen is in solution with about a pint of water per 500 calories. In contrast, fat can be stored in any quantity, contains only 20 percent water and equates to 3500 calories per pound. Thus a calorie counting diet that lowers glycogen results in rapid weight loss—and just as rapidly, puts weight back on. Twenty pounds of overweight fat is equal to 70,000 calories on top of over 100,000 calories of fat that a lean 175-pound man has in store. The T-Factor diet conserves lean body mass. With slower weight loss on the T-Factor diet, you are finally in control, fit, and full of energy.

Because appetite/hunger is dictated by glycogen stores, it is possible to gain weight and still be hungry when fat foods are eaten. Most snack foods are 65 percent fat. A 240-calorie candy bar is about 80 calories carbohydrate and 160 calories of fat. Now apply this to a meal. First, dieting does not mean skipping meals. Eating prevents your being overly hungry. Second, if you need to replenish 500 calories, do it mainly with carbohydrates. Fat does not take away hunger ... it just makes you fat.

The mysterious "set point" or appestat discussed in many diet books is a myth. Each person has "a range of adaptability within which permanent changes in diet and exercise operate with a certain ease and convenience, ... of 50 to 75 pounds" (Katahn, 1989, p. 228).

After skipping a meal, or meals, one tends to overeat. Sight, smells, conviviality—many variables affect the appetite. The most potent is glycogen stores. Katahn shows how easy it is to overeat the fat that comes along when needed carbohydrate would fulfill the hunger.

Katahn postulates that "the differences in the way your body metabolizes fat compared with protein and carbohydrates are so great that, except for the small minority who suffer from some metabolic abnormality, you can't get fat except by eating fat" (Katahn, 1989, p. 17).

However, there must be far more people than Katahn believes exist whose metabolism leads to hyperinsulinism. I presume that members of the overweight population who have gained weight rather slowly with aging can profitably follow the Katahn diet. I also presume that those who tended to be overweight from a young age, who have dieted often and have failed as often, these, the most frustrated dieters, will greet the Zone as their savior.

As convincingly as Katahn postulates the eating of carbohydrates vis-à-vis lipids, Montignac, in the next chapter, shows that high glycemic carbohydrates trigger fat retention. The glycemic index is ignored by Katahn.

Katahn's diet (1989) preceded the Pyramid Diet; it preceded also the wide knowledge of glycemic index, which makes these starch-based diets tough on us Paleolithic types. Prior to 1992, the USDA (United States Department of Agriculture) diet was based on the Four Food Groups:

- Milk and Milk Products
- Meat, Fish
- Breads, Grains
- Vegetables, Fruits

Therapeutic diets had proscribed saturated fats for many years; the USDA Pyramid Diet was a long time coming. An excellent description is given in the Oct. 1992 *Consumer Reports* article, "Eating Right, It's Easier Than You Think." The Pyramid graphically pictures the daily eating suggestions.

| | | |
|---|---|---|
| **Base** | 6 to 11 servings | Bread, Cereal, Rice, Pasta |
| **Second Level** | 3 to 5 servings | Vegetables, and |
| | 2 to 4 servings | Fruit |
| **Third Level** | 2 to 3 servings | Milk, Yogurt, Cheese, and |
| | 2 to 3 servings | Meat, Poultry, Fish, Dried Beans, Nuts |
| **Top** | Use sparingly | Fats, Oil, Sweets |

The *Consumer Reports* article goes further to present a consensus report of the 68 answering (out of 94 polled) nutrition experts, members of Federal Advisory Boards, and the like. Dissenting comments were not provided, yet

the glycemic index described in the next chapter was known. Major conclusions are:
- 25% of calories or less from fat (as near as I could see, total calories average 2250 which would equate to 62.5 fat grams).
- 7 or more servings of vegetables and fruits daily.
- No more than 3 three-ounce servings of red meat weekly.
- Dietary cholesterol 200 to 300 milligrams or lower daily.
- No more than 7 percent of calories to be saturated fat (meat and cheese fat).
- Fish 2 or more times per week.
- Protein, about 65 grams daily, which becomes 12 percent of a 2250 calorie diet. This amount is presented as normal in 1992.
- At least 6 servings of starches daily, getting more than half of daily calories as carbohydrate.
- Cut sugars from present 11% to 5% of total calories.

It is interesting to read "How Good is Mr. Hurley's Diet" by Francis Bello in December 1959 *Fortune Magazine*. Roy Hurley, then president of Curtis Wright Corporation, had personally consulted with the nation's known diet and nutrition experts. His consensus state-of-the-art diet has a greater comparison to the Zone Diet in Chapter Five. But the premise for it—obtaining low cholesterol and a healthy heart—is the basis of the 1992 Pyramid Diet. In fact, listing the no-nos would be totally similar for any diet discussed in this book.

DO NOT EAT:
1. Pastries, pies, cookies, cakes, muffins, doughnuts, unless prepared at home using corn or cottonseed oil or special margarine as the only source of fat.

2. Bacon, sausages, corned beef, luncheon meats.
3. Whole milk, ice cream, chocolate candy, butter, ordinary margarine, sour or sweet cream, lard, hard cheese, cream cheese, or creamed cottage cheese.
4. Gravy or salad dressings unless made with corn oil, cottonseed oil, mayonnaise, or special margarine.
5. Cream soups.
6. Potato chips, popcorn, and other fried foods, unless prepared using oils as instructed.

(Bello, Dec. 1959, *Fortune*, p. 7)

So each diet lays claim to the same happy result and all diets listed in this book will function to lose weight. *Of course, it is the ease of the regimen and how it leaves you feeling that determine its ultimate success.*

What went on between 1959 and 1992? Some vital new knowledge for us Paleolithic types was the "glycemic index."

# 3

# THE LOW GLYCEMIC DIET

*Dine Out and Lose Weight*
Michel Montignac
(Montignac USA, 1991)
***Obesity: Gluttony or Genes***
Edgar Gordon (Postgraduate Medicine, June 1969)

The superiority of complex carbohydrates over simple sugar has been de rigueur for years, recommended by nutritionists for diabetics and for Americans as a whole by the pyramid diet. Supposedly the molecular structure of starches such as pasta, rice, and breadstuffs, being more complex than sugar, sucrose, made them "complex" and sugar "simple." Thus they were digested more slowly and did not overstimulate the production of insulin. This seemingly logical assumption is in our national psyche. It is very wrong.

Actually, a carbohydrate's molecular complexity plays little role in the speed at which glucose is freed and assimilated by the body. Research has now provided the "glycemic index" to compare the blood sugar response versus elapsed time for all of the carbohydrate foods. Tables of "good" or "bad" are presented in this chapter.

Michel Montignac formulated his 1987 French best-selling book, *Dine Out and Lose Weight*, central to these facts. Its essence is this: when a "bad" carbohydrate is ingested with fat, the excess insulin produces an abnormal retention of blood fatty acids. Meals should, therefore, be fat free if average carbohydrates are eaten or if they are lipid/protein, eaten with low glycemic carbohydrates. Three hours should elapse between a carbohydrate meal and a lipid/protein one. The "rules" are easy to learn and follow; hunger does not result since overproduced insulin does not lower blood sugar.

According to Montignac (1991):
- Never mix bad carbohydrates with lipids in the same meal. Examine tables pages 27 and 28 for bad carbohydrates and see explanation following.
- Avoid carbohydrate/lipids; milk chocolate, avocados, hazelnuts, etc.
- Eliminate sugar completely from your diet.
- Never eat refined flours.
- Eat only whole wheat or bran bread made with unbleached flour and only at breakfast.
- Eliminate potatoes, especially fried.
- Eliminate white rice.
- Eat fruit alone on an empty stomach with skin, if possible.
- Give up all alcohol: cocktails, beer, wine, liqueurs (add red wine on maintenance diet).
- Avoid strong coffee; get into the habit of drinking decaffeinated.
- Never skip a meal. Eat three meals a day at the same time if possible.
- Take time eating. Chew well.

- Wait three hours after a carbohydrate meal, like breakfast, before eating any lipids.
- Eat a lot of fibers: lettuce, leeks, asparagus, artichokes, eggplant, etc.
- Definitely abandon bad eating habits typical to the United States; all sandwiches, hamburgers, hot dogs, candy and sodas, chemically processed sauces, i.e. ketchup, salad dressing, mayonnaise; popcorn and potato chips.
- Avoid snacking.
- Reduce saturated fat consumption.
- Consume monounsaturated (olive oil) and polyunsaturated fats.
- Eat more vegetables; lentils, beans, et al.
- Eat more fish—minimum of 11 ounces weekly.
- Eat fibers regularly—fruits, vegetables.
- Strive for sufficient intake of vitamins A, E, C, and selenium.

Ingesting excess carbohydrate together with lipids (fat) causes weight gain in people who produce too much insulin. Montignac postulates that fat people are, or have a tendency to be, hypoglycemic. **A vicious cycle of excess carbohydrates triggers too much insulin which triggers low blood sugar which triggers hunger and produces the fat person who can only rage at those, not afflicted, who grandly pronounce, *"just count calories."***

The **glycemic index** for a certain food is a ratio of hyperglycemic potential caused by that food compared to glucose which is rated 100 percent. The higher the blood sugar increase induced by the tested carbohydrate, the higher the glycemic index. It is the rate of entry of a carbohydrate into the blood stream *(see Figure 1)*.

The crux of Montignac's diet is to eat only low glycemic index carbohydrates with lipids. And his great con-

**FIGURE 1**

Curves demonstrating response to glucose leading to Glycemic Index Ratings (Source: Montignac, 1991, p. 246).

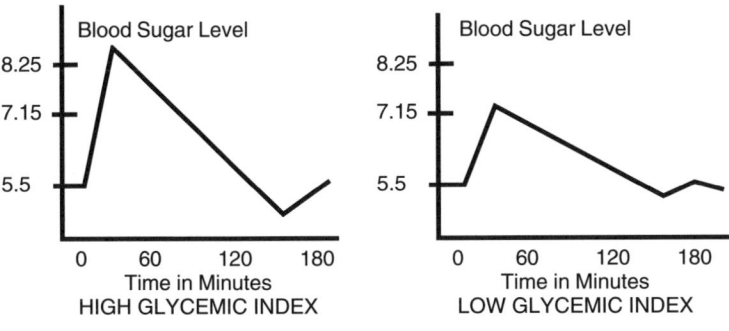

tribution is the classification of "good" and "bad" carbohydrates. *(Study tables on pages 27-31. Reprinted by permission from* Dine Out and Lose Weight *by Michel Montignac).*

"The Starch Reality," an article authored by Bob Barnett in the Sept. 1995 *Men's Journal,* discusses a *New York Times* article which lumped pasta and other "complex" carbohydrates with sugar, and quotes a spokesperson of the Tufts Human Nutrition Research Center:

> The Times *pointed to starchy foods like pasta, rice and potatoes—even white bread—as culprits in making you fat, but what they failed to tell you is that starchy foods are complex carbohydrates which are good for regulating insulin levels and weight. Unlike simple carbohydrates, like sugar and alcohol which are absorbed quickly by the body, complex carbohydrates are digested and absorbed slowly in the small intestine.*

Although the glycemic index was known in 1995, it was not well known enough, and it still isn't. My earliest reference is in the 1986 book by Roy Walford, The 120-Year Diet. He writes, "For many years it was assumed *(without actual testing of the assumption)* [italics added] that complex carbohydrates ... or starches such as rice and potatoes were slowly digested and absorbed, causing only a small rise in blood sugar, whereas simple carbohydrates like table sugar were readily digested and rapidly absorbed" (Walford, 1986, p. 209). Walford cites research of 1977, 1981, and 1984 and goes on to say that most people break down complex carbohydrates to simple ones almost immediately. The table on page 27 shows that the actual effect of carbohydrate foods is far different than expected. Regular sugar is not as bad as white bread or mashed potatoes or beer. This, however, does not make sugar good.

> Adelle Davis equated starches to sugar back in 1954, telling us that the effect of a high carbohydrate meal was to increase blood sugar, calling for more insulin, which would withdraw the blood sugar—i.e. describing the vicious cycle perfectly. She advocated a breakfast of moderate protein with a small amount of "sugar" and fat to give sustained energy. We have known this for years, and finally the research on glycemic index proves it.

Montignac says a great deal more about cholesterol and fiber and saturated fat and sugar. Tellingly, he points out, "You will see that once your system has completely absorbed your fat surplus, you will be able to reintegrate lipids containing bad carbohydrates into your diet, as long as you do it prudently" (Montignac, 1991, p. 65).

As you read on, it is important to remember that the Montignac Diet postulates a great deal of green vegetable, low glycemic carbohydrate, and that the Barry Sears Zone Diet provides a measure for this—4 parts carbohydrate to 3 parts protein. Unfortunately, the critics, either as a misreading or deliberately it does seem, lump these diets in with meat-only diets that do cut down carbohydrates to a level that causes an abnormal fat metabolism, termed ketosis. In ketosis, organic chemicals, or ketones, are formed which must be lost through urination. This is a controversial diet procedure that most diet professionals malign.

These high meat diets have been with us for some time. Dr. Richard Mackarness published *Eat Fat and Grow Slim* in 1959 and quotes William Bunting, who in London in 1862 weighed 202 pounds at the age of 66, as stating that he went down stairways backward. Bunting wrote the first meat-only diet book, stating he ate "joynts" of meat only and achieved slenderness. Dr. Robert Atkins wrote the *Diet Revolution* in 1972. But now finally we have the glycemic index which revolutionizes the concept of complex carbohydrates. And we have the Zone Diet which provides a healthy proportion of carbohydrates which prevent ketosis while providing the fiber, minerals, and vitamins of a healthy diet.

Over a period of six months in 1969, I lost 39 pounds following a precursor of the Atkins' diet. Probably 90 percent of the calories were lipid protein, yet cholesterol dropped from 296 to 140.

In June of 1969, Dr. Edgar Gordon of the University of Wisconsin published a paper in *Post Graduate Medicine* that corroborates the work of Montignac. Dr. Gordon felt that obesity may be a true metabolic defect. There are three anomalies: defective glucose metabolism, hyperinsulinism, and water retention. He says:

> *The normal person burns the carbohydrate that he eats, whereas the obese converts large amounts of it into fat and stores the fat. This is a kind of diabetes in that it is a defect in carbohydrate metabolism.*
>
> *All obese persons have a form of hyperinsulinism. The insulin response to a glucose challenge has been as much as 10 times greater in an obese individual than in a normal one.* **Figure 2** *shows that insulin response following a glucose challenge in obese non-diabetics and diabetics and in thin*

*nondiabetics and diabetics. The total response of the obese person is much greater, indicating an overreaction of the pancreatic islets and consequently an overproduction of insulin.*

*Hyperinsulinism in the obese is due to an excessive amount of adipose tissue. When an obese subject's weight is reduced to normal, his glucose tolerance curve and insulin output become normal **(see Figure 3)**. As far as we know, hyperinsulinism is not a cause of obesity but rather a response to it.*

*How do hyperinsulinism and defective carbohydrate metabolism fit together? The oversized fat cells in the obese store an excessive amount of fat, causing an intense resistance to the basic physiologic action of insulin. When the size of the fat cells reverts to normal, insulin sensitivity becomes normal. This metabolic defect is also found in obese diabetics.* (Gordon, 1969, pp. 98, 99).

**FIGURE 2**

Following a glucose challenge, the hyper-response to insulin is obvious in the obese subjects. (Reprinted by permission. *Post Graduate Medicine,* Gordon, June, 1969, McGraw Hill Co.)

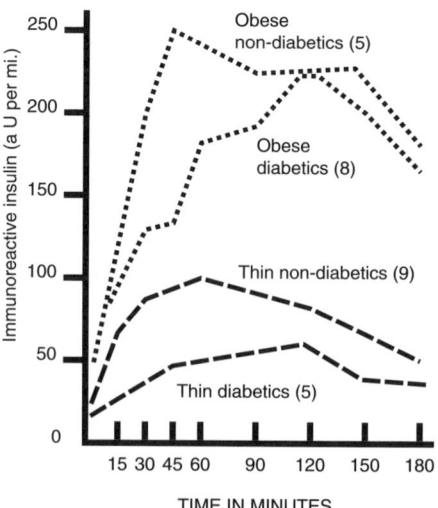

**FIGURE 3**

Glucose tolerance tests in a maturity-onset diabetic show the effect of weight reduction on blood glucose and serum levels. Dotted lines indicate levels before weight reduction from 20 percent over to 5 percent under ideal weight. Broken lines show levels after weight reduction. (Reprinted by permission. *Post Graduate Medicine,* Gordon, June, 1969, McGraw Hill Co.)

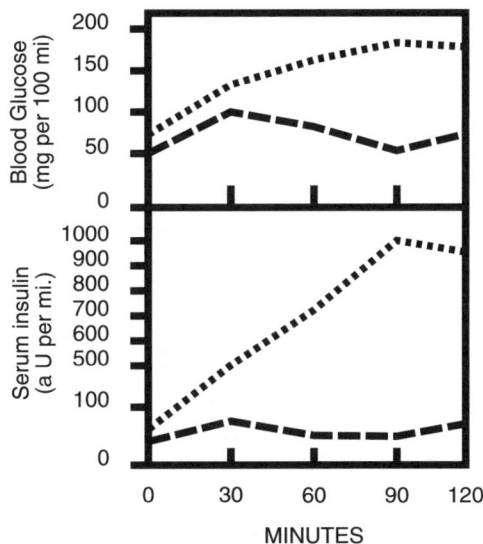

The key factors here are the clinical verification of the efficacy of the Montignac-Sears diet and the fact that once the obese lose mass, they become normal in insulin response. Cholesterol levels, if elevated when obese, will also normalize. Cholesterol has become a shibboleth in nutritionist thinking. Reduction of lipids may lower cholesterol in thin persons; reduction of high glycemic carbohydrate will lower the weight of the obese, which returns cholesterol to normal. National death comparisons for heart disease show that those countries that are large consumers of hypoglycemic foods such as sugar, white flour, potatoes, and beer are severalfold worse than the fresh fruit, vegetable, and olive oil countries. There is much evidence to show that starch and sugar are the greatest culprits. *(See bar chart in Figure 4.)*

**FIGURE 4**

Death rates for coronoary heart disease in 1985 by country, men and women, 35-74 years of age, per 100,000 population.

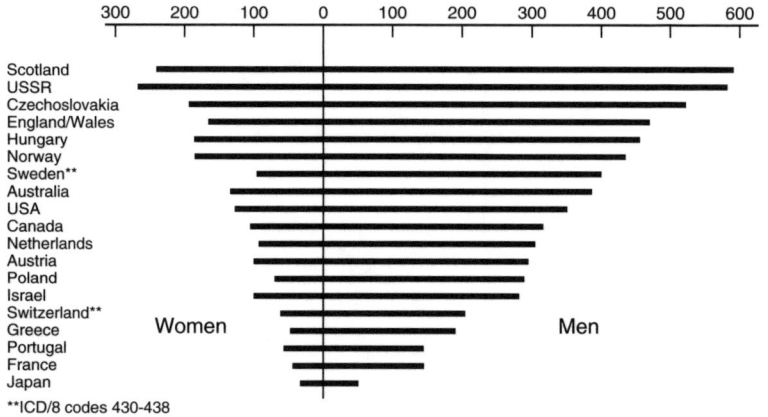

Source: WHO, Health Statistics Annual, Montagnac. Reprinted by permission of World Health Organization.

## TABLE 3
## Glycemic Index for Different Carbohydrates

| | | | |
|---|---|---|---|
| Maltose | 110 | Whole wheat bread | 50 |
| Glucose | 100 | Oatmeal | 50 |
| White bread | 95 | Whole wheat pasta | 45 |
| Instant mashed potatoes | 95 | Fresh white beans | 40 |
| Highly refined sugar | 95 | Whole rye bread | 40 |
| Honey, jam | 90 | Green peas | 40 |
| Cornflakes | 85 | Whole grain cereal | 35 |
| Carrots | 85 | Multigrain bread | 35 |
| White sugar | 75 | Milk products | 35 |
| Corn | 70 | Fresh fruits | 35 |
| French bread | 70 | Wild rice | 35 |
| White rice | 70 | Lentils | 30 |
| Beets | 70 | Chick peas | 30 |
| Cookies | 70 | Milk | 30 |
| Boiled potatoes | 70 | Dried beans | 30 |
| Pasta | 65 | Dark chocolate | 22 |
| Sherbet | 65 | Fructose | 20 |
| Banana | 60 | Soy | 15 |
| Grapes | 60 | Peanuts | 15 |
| Bran cereal | 50 | Green vegetables | 15 |
| Brown rice | 50 | | |

It is imperative to keep in mind that chemical processing of foods increase their glycemic index. (Cornflakes-85, Corn-70 ... instant Mashed potatoes-95, Boiled potatoes-70). (Source: Montignac, 1991, p. 246.)

The results are unexpected. Beer and rice cakes (not shown) are both 110. Remember that high glycemic foods trigger excessive insulin and should not be eaten with fat. Excessive insulin lowers blood sugar, which is metabolized to fat retained in the body, and increases hunger, thus repeating the process upon the almost inevitable act of eating. In the absence of fat and excessive carbohydrate calories, the body burns retained fat-stores for energy. Thus you lose weight and yet are not hungry except at meal intervals.

## TABLE 4
## Classification of Carbohydrates

| EXCELLENT (less than 15 glycemic index) | GOOD (less than 50 glycemic index) | BAD (over 50 glycemic index) | |
|---|---|---|---|
| Alfalfa sprouts | Beans | Alcohol (especially distilled) | Potatoes |
| Artichokes | Bran | | Potato starch |
| Bamboo shoots | Brown rice | Bleached flour (french bread, rolls) | Quiche |
| Bell peppers | Chick peas | | Refined cereals (corn flakes, puffed rice) |
| Broccoli | Chocolate (with more than 60% cocoa) | Cakes (made with white flour and sugar) | |
| Cabbage | | | Semolina, Couscous |
| Cauliflower | Fruits | | |
| Celery | Lentils | Carrots | Soft drinks |
| Cucumbers | Wheat germ | Chocolate (with less than 60% cocoa) | Sugars (beet, brown) |
| Eggplant | Whole cereals (wheat, oats, barley, millet, etc.) | | Sweet potatoes |
| Hearts of palm | | | |
| Leeks | | Cookies, Croissants | Sweets |
| Lettuce | Whole wheat bread | | White rice |
| Mushrooms | Whole wheat flour | Corn | |
| Radishes | Whole wheat pasta | Corn starch | |
| Salsify | | Honey | |
| Soy beans | | Jams, Jellies | |
| Spinach | | Maple syrup | |
| Split peas | | Molasses | |
| Squash | | Pasta | |
| String beans | | Pizza | |
| Tomatoes | | | |
| Turnips | | | |

Source: Montignac, 1991, p. 45.

There is excellent corroboration of this data in the research quoted in the *Modern Nutrition in Health and Disease "Handbook"* following these tables and in the *Zone* books. Almost unlimited amounts of excellent rated carbohydrates may be eaten.

## TABLE 5
## Classification of Foods As Macronutrients

| PROTEIN/FAT* | CARBOHYDRATES | CARBOHYDRATE/FAT | FIBERS |
|---|---|---|---|
| Beef | Alcohol | Almonds | Artichokes |
| Butter | Beans | Avocado | Asparagus |
| Cheeses | Bread | Cashews | Bell peppers |
| Crab | Chick peas | Chestnuts | Cabbage |
| Cold cuts | Cookies | Chocolate | Egg plant |
| Eggs | Corn | Coconut | Endives |
| Fish | Couscous | Egg noodles | Leeks |
| Lamb | Dry fruit | Hazelnuts | Lettuce |
| Lobster | Flour | Liver | Mushrooms |
| Olive Oil | Fruit | Milk | Salsify |
| Peanut oil | Honey | Olives | Sauerkraut |
| Pork | Lentils | Oysters | Spinach |
| Poultry | Pasta | Peanuts | Squash |
| Prawns | Peas | Scallops | String beans |
| Rabbit | Potatoes | Soy flour | Tomatoes |
| Shrimp | Rice | Walnuts | Turnips |
| Veal | Semolina | Water chestnuts | |
| | Sugar | | |
| | Tapioca | | |

*All foods in this column (except butter and oils) contain protein
Source: Montignac, 1991, p. 44.

> *In view of the many differences in man, it would be surprising if the chemical machinery governing the use of energy containing fuels were the same in all. Perhaps some persons have more efficient "engines" than others. Overweight would be a constant problem in these individuals. An average intake of food would provide them with an oversupply of energy, which would be stored in adipose tissue.* —Gordon (1969, p. 95)

## TABLE 6
## Classification of Allowed Foods
## for Montignac Weight Loss Diet

| APPETIZERS | ENTREES | VEGETABLES | DESSERTS |
|---|---|---|---|
| Asparagus | Crayfish | Bell peppers | Cheeses |
| Crab | Cold cuts | Broccoli | Cottage Cheese |
| Celery | Eggs | Cabbage | Yogurt |
| Cold cuts | Fish (all) | Cauliflower | (unsweetened) |
| Eggs | Lobster | Celery | |
| Leeks | Meat | Eggplant | |
| Lobster | (except liver) | Endives | |
| Mushrooms | Poultry | Fennel | |
| Mussels | Rabbit | Leeks | |
| Radishes | | Lettuce: | |
| Salads: | SEASONINGS | *Iceberg* | |
| *Cauliflower* | Béarnaise sauce | *Red leaf* | |
| *Cucumber* | Butter | *Spinach* | |
| *Endive* | Garlic | Mushrooms | |
| *String Beans* | Herbs | Sauerkraut | |
| *Tomato* | Margarine | Sorrel | |
| Salmon, Fresh | Olive oil | Spinach | |
| Salmon, Smoked | Onions | Squash | |
| Sardines | Peanut oil | String Beans | |
| Tuna | Pepper | Tomatoes | |
| | Salt | Turnips | |
| | Shallots | | |

Source, Montignac, 1991, p. 229.

Remember that this table of foods for weight loss and the one following for weight maintenance are based on French gastronomy. They will give you the idea or principle of the food selections. Appendix 2 provides a Primer of Optimal Nutrition. The *Zone* books provide a convenient "block" method to judge this information with closely similar classification data.

## TABLE 7
## Classification of Allowed Foods
## for Montignac Weight Maintenance Diet

| APPETIZERS | ENTREES | VEGETABLES | DESSERTS |
|---|---|---|---|
| Avocado* | Cold cuts | Bell peppers | Blackberries* |
| Celery | Crayfish | Broccoli | Cheeses |
| Cold cuts | Eggs | Cabbage | Chocolate |
| Crab | Fish (all) | Cauliflower | mousse* |
| Crayfish | Lobster | Celery | Cottage Cheese |
| Eggs | Meat (all) | Eggplant | Raspberries* |
| Foie Gras* | Poultry | Endives | Strawberries |
| Hearts of Palm | Rabbit | Fennel | Strawberry |
| Leeks | | Leeks | shortcake |
| Lettuce | **SEASONINGS** | Lettuce: | Sorbet: |
| Lobster | | *Iceberg* | Raspberry gratin* |
| Mussels | Béarnaise sauce | *Red leaf* | Strawberry |
| Prawns | Butter | *Spinach* | Yogurt |
| Radishes | Garlic | Mushrooms | |
| Salads: | Herbs | Salsify | |
| *Cauliflower* | Margarine | Sauerkraut | |
| *Cucumber* | Mayonnaise | Sorrel | |
| *Endive* | Mustard* | Spinach | |
| *Mushroom* | Olive oil | Squash | |
| *String Beans* | Onions | String Beans | |
| *Tomato* | Peanut oil | Tomatoes | |
| *Walnut* | Pepper | Turnips | |
| Salmon, Fresh | Salt | | |
| Salmon, Smoked | Shallots | | |
| Sardines | | | |
| Scallops | | | |
| Shrimp | | | |
| Tuna | | | |

*Note: The foods marked with an asterisk are allowed if they are eaten in moderate amounts. Refrain from eating more than two per meal. According to the method, anything not listed should be avoided, but certain "discrepancies" are possible.

Source: Montignac, 1991, p. 230.

Dining out and at parties is made enjoyable following the Montignac precepts. You may not "lose" weight, but you will hold your own!

A medical school compendium, *Modern Nutrition In Health and Disease*, 8th Edition, 1994 by Shils, Olson, and Shike does provide technical verification of the glycemic index and the concepts of insulin and glucose control, proof of the theorems of Montignac and of Sears (following in Chapter Five).

The Glycemic Index topic on pages 596 and 597 is reprinted with permission:

*Because many factors in foods may influence their rates of digestion and glycemic responses, and because most of these factors are not listed in food tables and many have nothing to do with food composition, it is not possible to predict the physiologic effect of a food on the basis of its chemical composition. Therefore, the glycemic index was developed as an index of the physiologic effect of foods to supplement information on chemical composition. It was reasoned that such information may allow a better understanding of the effects of carbohydrate foods and aid in the selection of appropriate foods for therapeutic diets. The glycemic index is defined as the blood glucose response to a 50g available carbohydrate portion of a food expressed as a percentage of the response to the same amount of carbohydrate from a standard food, which has been either glucose or white bread.*

The authors go on to cite research papers which show the clinical relevance of low glycemic index foods:
- To reduce blood lipids
- To reduce insulin secretion
- To improve blood glucose control
- To enhance dietary satiety.

The table of glycemic index in relation to white bread is in general agreement with the Montignac data presented herein. A second table compares digestive rates of common foods ... that legumes produce about one-third the concentration of blood sugars at three hours after ingestion than do starches such as white bread, rice, or potatoes. The authors say, "As data accumulate, it should be possible to select diets on the basis of rates of digestion to achieve the desired physiologic and metabolic effects" (Shils, Olson & Shike, 1994, p. 596).

Central to the Montignac diet, and to those of us with Paleolithic genes, is the concept of glycemic index, which is the rate at which the glucose metabolized from a carbohydrate enters the blood stream. This stimulates insulin, which, according to Barry Sears, is the greatest indicator of heart problems (Sears, 1995, p. 137). The insulin causes the glucose to metabolize to fat, and at the same time, prevents body fat from being used for energy. Hunger results, and eating repeats the obesity cycle. For me, glycemic index was a revelation; it explained so much. Yet the usual nutrition experts have been silent, and therefore the media have also.

Because of it, the Montignac diet is effective. Particularly will the Montignac diet function as a life eating pattern where more calories may be eaten. A primer of nutrition is provided in the next chapter. How can you be a hunter-gatherer in our modern supermarkets? Then in Chapter Five, "The Zone" quantifies the macronutrients and provides a precise pattern of wellness derived from diet.

# 4

# THE TRAINING TABLE

***The Balancing Act, Nutrition and Weight Guide***
Georgia G. Kostas, MPH, RD
(Balancing Act, 1993)
***Homocysteine Revolution***
Dr. Kilmer S. McCully (Keats Publishing, 1997)
***Optimal Nutrition***
The Cooper Clinic Nutrition Program, Georgia G. Kostas, et al.
*This tipsheet available at (972) 239-7223*
***The Complete Book of Food Counts***
Corinne T. Netzer (Dell Publishing, 1997)

In this chapter we discuss the maintenance diet after a desirable weight level has been attained, making note of how the diet patterns of Katahn and Montignac fit Paleolithic nutrition and how they lead to the Zone.

Here, we will provide a guide to basic nutrition and define terms that appear on food containers and in the media, and refer you to the books listed above. We are particularly pleased to present Georgia Kostas' Cooper Clinic Optimal Nutrition Tipsheet in Appendix 1.

**MEAT.** The human body is continually wearing out and being renewed. Many thousands of different proteins are synthesized, usually from meat sources, and some, the essential amino acids, must be ingested. Protein cannot be stored in the body *but must be replenished daily* to keep in "balance," since some protein is being broken down each day.

The U.S. Food and Nutrition Board recommends 0.26 grams protein intake per pound body weight for adults, twice this much for growing children, and higher for infants (Pauling, 1988, p. 27). The same source indicates that the U.S. Senate Select Committee on Nutrition and Human Needs recommends an average of 75 grams daily for a diet of 2500 calories (Pauling, 1988, p. 33). For a person weighing 200 pounds, such as myself, 0.26 grams protein means a daily requirement of 52 grams. Since 2500 calories is about right for me, and the Select Committee tells me 75 grams, I venture an opinion that the 52-gram figure is based on life support and the 75-gram figure is for robust living, just as 60 milligrams used to be the RDA (Recommended Daily Allowance) of vitamin C to prevent scurvy and now 2000 to 4000 to 6000 milligrams is recommended for robust health.

In her nutrition column of November 1996, Liz Applegate, Ph.D., the nutrition director of *Runner's World Magazine*, stated that the RDA of protein for sedentary people should be 0.36 grams per pound—for me, 73 daily grams, corresponding to the Pauling RDA. She goes on to indicate that active people, in this case runners, need much more—between 0.50 and 0.72 grams per pound—for me, 100 to 145 daily protein grams. The caveat is that protein sources should be carefully selected to eliminate fat—which is hard to do, as we shall see. We discuss protein at length because it is central to our food needs, particularly in the Zone diet of the next chapter. Paleolithic man, with 3000 calories daily, ingested 250 grams of protein!

Appendix One provides the fat and cholesterol content of typical protein/lipid sources. Our goal is to select meats that minimize saturated fat so that the P:S ratio, polyunsaturated fat to saturated, is about 60:40. *As protein cannot be stored in the body nor can the essential amino acids be synthesized, these are both a daily need.* Wild meat met these daily needs; today we should tend towards most fowl, fish, and very lean red meat.

Both the Katahn and Montignac diets can comply if saturated fat is minimized and quantities of protein are "normal," but amounts are not specified in the diets. We will see that the Zone diet in Chapter Five provides a discrete quantity of protein, as well as fat and carbohydrate, for each person and activity level, thus removing ambiguities.

**PLANT FOODS.** Starch is the principal carbohydrate food, found in all fruits, vegetables, and grains. Many fruits and vegetables also contain glucose and fructose as well as ordinary sugar. Humankind has been accustomed to metabolizing/burning glucose digested from starchy foods for millions of years. Starch is digested by the saliva and stomach juices to form glucose which passes through the walls of the intestines into the blood stream. Glucose present in foods or broken down from sucrose proceeds in the same fashion.

Roots, beans, nuts, tubers, fruits, flowers, and gums made up the gatherers' diet, amounting to 3 to 5 pounds of rough plant foods daily. Refined grains (even grindstones) were unknown. Primitive food processing retained most of the plant fiber.

Grains defined the age of agriculture which provided concentrated calories for its burgeoning population at the expense of protein nutrition. The resulting decrease in body size has only now been made up by today's plentiful food supply. Katahn recommends unlimited grains which Montignac bans as high glycemic, the exception being whole grains which still should not be eaten with lipids.

**SUGARS.** *When simple sugar, sucrose, is eaten, it is broken down into equal parts of glucose and fructose.* Natural fructose is the "sugar" found in fruit. According to Linus Pauling, humankind was accustomed to digesting only about 8 grams per day of fructose but is now deluged by modern sugar consumption of 75 grams daily coming from sugar sucrose. On average, modern Americans obtain about 20 percent of their calories from simple sugar, about 120 pounds per capita per year! This compares to

> *I believe that if people were to avoid sucrose—never spoon out a spoonful of sugar from the sugar bowl onto anything, avoid sweet desserts except when you're a guest somewhere, avoid buying foods that say "sugar" as one of the contents—they could cut down on the incidence of disease and increase life expectancy.*
>
> *Do not drink soft drinks. The common 12-ounce cola drink contains 8½ teaspoons of sugar. If you were to drink two a day and eat the ordinary American diet, your sucrose intake would be 155 pounds per year.*
>
> —Linus Pauling (from a speech given at Cal Tech, August 1979)

four pounds annually in the year 1800 and much less in prehistory when honey was the sole concentrated sweetener. Sugar, today ubiquitous in cold drinks, ice cream, candy, and desserts (along with chemicals and saturated fats), has been lessened in both diets, more so by Montignac.

So 50 percent of sugar as glucose proceeds directly to the blood stream. The other 50 percent, as fructose, or "fruit sugar," is further metabolized to glucose and acetate. This slows down metabolism so that fruits in general have a lower glycemic index than starches. Even so-called simple sugar (sucrose) has a lower glycemic index than many refined starches. It is not as "simple" as many nutritionists tell us since it is half fructose. Investigators point out that whole fruit with fibers is much healthier than juice since digestion is slowed. Montignac tells us to eat fruit alone 20 minutes before breakfast or as a snack.

**FAT.** Triglycerides are the fats found in food and the blood stream. Fat provides 9 calories per gram. Carbohydrate and protein each provide 4 calories per gram.

A proportion of animal fat and fat in dairy products is "saturated" because the molecules are "closed" or filled with hydrogen. Olive and fish oils, salmon, and nuts (natural peanut butter) are termed mono-unsaturated since the molecules have an "opening" and will permit the manufacture of necessary hormones. Vegetable fats and oils used in salad dressings are polyunsaturated fats, having two or more "openings" in their molecular make-up. If these openings are "filled," i.e., hydrogenated, the food product will be "solid" and creamy and have long shelf life, but lose its value in producing good hormones. Essential fatty acids, which are in daily need as they cannot be synthesized, are found in unsaturated fats.

A good rule of thumb is that fats that are solid at room temperature are saturated, those that are liquid at room temperature but solidify in the refrigerator are mono-unsaturated, and those that are still liquid in the refrigerator are polyunsaturated. Saturated fats are termed "bad," unsaturated fats "good!" Unsaturated fat protects against arteriosclerosis, but can oxidize. Adelle Davis advised 40 years ago not to eat hydrogenated fat and to throw out rancid fat.

Research on the role of fat and fat types is ongoing, especially mono-unsaturated fats. Olive oil, which is mono-unsaturated is vital to the heart-healthy Mediterranean diet. The current aim of the American Heart Association is to have equal proportions of the three fat types. The listing of fat and cholesterol content of meats and dairy products in Appendix 1 gives guidelines—and some surprising data. Meats and dairy products are quite satisfactory, if quantities are reasonable.

|  | FAT PERCENT | |
|---|---|---|
|  | UNSATURATED | SATURATED |
| Lean beef | 56 | 44 |
| Lean pork | 56 | 44 |
| Fish | 96 | 4 |
| Cheddar cheese | 40 | 60 |
| Whole milk | 37 | 63 |
| Ice cream | 55 | 45 |
| Butter | 50 | 50 |
| Tub Margarine | 82 | 18 |
| Vegetable oil | 100 | 0 |

**CHOLESTEROL.** Cholesterol is a crystalline fatty alcohol, an organic compound found in cell membranes, and is necessary for production of many hormones. It is produced in animal cells and not found in plants. Humans synthesize about 3500 milligrams per day. It is vital for all body tissues. In this book, we discuss foods and diets that may lower blood levels of cholesterol, which in turn should lessen fatty deposits in the blood vessels.

A blood profile will give amounts of fat, triglycerides, and cholesterol of various types. These products must be transported in the blood stream by protein carriers termed lipoproteins. HDL is high density lipoprotein, LDL low density lipoprotein.

It is accepted today that serum cholesterol levels are raised by total fat intake and lowered by the polyunsaturated to saturated fat ratio. Early man ingested somewhat more cholesterol than today's average. Wild game meat had much less fat, relatively less saturated. Cholesterol is in connective tissue. With today's hunter-gatherers, cholesterol intake ranges from 500 to 2000mg daily, well over today's recommended amounts of under 300mg, yet blood serum levels average 140 compared to 210 average in America, an indicator that many other factors of these primitive diets must be checked. The French diet is high in unsaturated fat, also high in total fat (cheeses), but low in simple sugar. French males have higher cholesterol on average than Americans, but much less heart disease (Clouatre, 1992, p. 131). Fat in the United States diet is epidemic, making up 42 percent of total diet calories. Two-thirds of this (28 percent) is saturated fat.

The Katahn diet counts fat grams. Montignac feels that more protein/fat may be eaten in the absence of high glycemic carbohydrate. Both suggest unsaturated fat.

There is convincing evidence that there is a correlation between the amount of cholesterol in the blood and the incidence of heart disease. The procedure recommended has been to decrease the eating of foods that contain cholesterol. However, according to Linus Pauling, there may be a more effective way to reduce cholesterol by

# Low-fat diet isn't best for some men

By Tim Friend
USA TODAY

PORTSMOUTH, N.H. — For many healthy men, eating a low-fat diet will not lower their cholesterol levels, and it may make them worse, new research suggests.

The findings, presented Monday at an American Heart Association (AHA) meeting, will help define who needs to make dietary sacrifices and who can abide by the adage "Everything in moderation."

"Not everybody is genetically programmed to go on a low-fat diet," says Ronald Krauss, University of California, Berkeley. In his studies, 200 healthy men went from a typical 30%-40% fat diet to a 20% fat diet. His findings:

▶ A third of the men had dramatic improvement on the 20% fat diet. These were men with normal levels of "bad" LDL cholesterol, but they had an onerous type called "small, dense LDL." They also had below-average "good" HDL cholesterol and high levels (above 200) of blood fats called triglycerides. These traits, associated with an increased risk of heart disease, are called Pattern B.

▶ A third of the men had ordinary LDL cholesterol, normal HDL and low levels (below 100) of triglycerides. These traits are called Pattern A. When these men adopted a 20% fat diet, they developed small, dense LDL, low HDL and high triglycerides.

▶ People in the middle, with triglycerides between 100 and 200, are not well-studied and could fit either profile.

Krauss says a third of all men fit Pattern B and a third are A. Among women, about a fifth are A and a fifth are B.

A test is being developed to show whether a person is A or B. In the meantime, Krauss says triglyceride levels provide a guide: above 200, eat a 20% fat diet; below 100, enjoy.

Copyright 1996 *USA Today*. Reprinted with permission.

means of changing nutrients that are known to be involved in the synthesis and destruction of cholesterol in our bodies. He cites research to show that sucrose, 50% of which becomes fructose, may be involved, since fructose metabolism produces acetate which is a raw material of cholesterol (Pauling, 1986, pp. 42, 74).

The July 16, 1996 *USA Today* ran the article, "Low Fat Diet Isn't Best for Some Men," containing information presented to the American Heart Association. What are we to conclude? One thing is that Linus Pauling is again right when he says that cholesterol in the food may not mean cholesterol in the blood stream. Another conclusion/suggestion is to have your blood lipids checked. A third evolves around a phrase in the article, "genetically programmed." This phrase implies the key point of this book—that we should emulate the natural eating patterns of our earliest ancestors.

Dallas Clouatre on cholesterol:
*The trick is to avoid blaming the messenger for the message. If high serum (blood) levels of LDL's in fact represent the body's attempt to compensate for a lack of antioxidants, then lowering cholesterol levels through heroic dietary measures and drug intervention is a false victory. If high cholesterol levels merely mark the presence of cholesterol-containing hormones associated with the body's response to stress, then the real answer is to slow down rather than to starve the body of the building blocks for hormones. Finally, if high LDL cholesterol levels, and especially high triglyceride levels, are the result of insulin-resistance and a diet high in sucrose, fructose, and refined carbohydrates and low in vitamins and minerals such as chromium, then the permanent solution is to stabilize blood sugar levels* (Clouatre, 1993, p. 132). (Author's note: Stabilizing blood sugar levels is precisely what is accomplished by the Zone diet.)

Barry Sears on cholesterol:
*Of course, no natural substance is entirely good or entirely bad. As an example, take cholesterol. Doctors like to describe different varieties of cholesterol with the terms good (high-density lipoproteins, or HDL) and bad (low-density*

*lipoproteins, or LDL). Well, as I said, there's no absolute good and there's no absolute bad in human physiology. Low-density lipoprotein (the carriers of bad cholesterol) are the molecular delivery trucks that transport the lipids, such as essential fatty acids and cholesterol, critical for cell growth. Without this bad cholesterol, you would die. It's when the balance of good and bad cholesterol becomes disturbed that the probability of cardiovascular trouble lurks ahead* (Sears, 1995, p. 34).

After all of these ambiguities, there is a new and perhaps revolutionary theory of blood vessel maladies. I had my first check of homocysteine levels in my blood profile of July, 1997. This is now regarded as a reliable indicator of cardiovascular disease, and it may indicate a watershed change in the belief that a high fat, high cholesterol intake is the primary cause of heart attacks and strokes. Homocysteine is a product of the normal metabolism of protein. It causes arteriosclerotic plaques by a direct affect of this amino acid on the cells and tissues of artery walls. High levels can be controlled with B-vitamins and folic acid. It is, of course, too early to cite many conclusions as to how this discovery will affect one's recommended diet. But it is one more reason to enter the Zone, where there is a balance between protein foods and green vegetables as excellent sources for folic acid and vitamins B6 and B12.

The *Homocysteine Revolution* is the book and life work of Dr. Kilmer S. McCully. It is a medical detective story that presents a unified theory which explains many of the empirical observations and quandaries of our present dietary and medical approaches to heart disease. You will forevermore "shop the outer aisles" after reading this book. It could well explain the long-term decrease in heart problems during the past thirty years as due to major improvements in the marketing of fresh vegetables and fruits, and why the "Mediterranean" diet is healthy for the heart.

Dr. McCully states that methionine, an amino acid found in all protein, would be minimized by eating less meat and that natural sources of vitamins B6, Folic Acid, and B12 should be augmented (McCully, 1997, p. 131). He suggests an optimal diet which would consist each day of 6 to 10 servings of raw, lightly cooked, or steamed vegetables or fruits; 2 to 3 servings of starchy vegetables and whole grains; and 1(!) small serving of meat, poultry, fish, eggs, or dairy products; also a bit of vegetable oil, such as olive, corn, or canola. A meat serving is 2 to 4 ounces (McCully, 1997, p. 156-162).

This is a low cholesterol diet more stringent with protein than the Pritikin Diet and is low glycemic. Criticisms of the Pritikin Diet center around its extraordinary restrictiveness, problems with total fiber content actually drawing minerals from the body, and raising triglyceride levels (Clouatre, 1995, p. 121). Will supplemental B-vitamins function to lower homocysteine levels in the Zone Diet which I consider to be protein adequate and low fat? Well, yes, my homocysteine level dropped 36 percent in six months with no change (except vitamin therapy) in my adherence to the Zone diet.

There must be balance! This is stressed by both Barry Sears and Linus Pauling. Here is an example. Too much polyunsaturated fat (and remember, we have a goal of increasing the ratio between unsaturated to saturated fat) can destroy the body's Vitamin E (Pauling, 1986, p. 155). This is a good reason to take Vitamin E and C, both antioxidants. But balance. You will read Pauling's advice in Chapter Eight, "Eat what you like, but not too much of any one food." Do not enter into radical unbalanced diets.

**FIBER.** Fiber ingestion from plant foods is essential to healthy digestion and waste passage. The rough plant foods of the Paleolithic provided protein and soluble and insoluble fiber, an estimated seven times more than today. The Montignac diet, with more attention to the unrefined grains and green vegetables, is better. It shuns high glycemic starches, sugars, and root vegetables. Add these when normal weight has been attained.

**SALT.** Potassium was about ten times more prevalent in the Paleolithic than salt; today it is the reverse. Here the Montignac diet, which proscribes refined cereals and snacks such as pretzels, is clearly better. While both diets recommend green vegetables, the Montignac bans more of the processed or canned foods which are high in sodium.

**CALCIUM AND TRACE MINERALS.** The hunter/gatherers met these needs in consuming a wide range of plant and animal life. Today it is estimated that only about 50 percent of the desired daily calcium intake of 1800mg is met, necessitating a supplement.

**VITAMIN C.** Early man is estimated to have ingested about 500mg of vitamin C from his daily three to five pounds of plant products. Today a supplement is needed.

**NUTRIENT DENSITY.** Foods of the past were bulky, fibrous, and dense in the *range* of nutrients, not calorically dense. A pound of venison contains 570 calories and 95g of protein. In contrast a pound of wieners contains 1400 calories and 57g of protein. An apple contains 80 percent fewer calories than the same weight of apple pie. This shows that modern foods contain more fat, less protein, and many more calories.

> *Choose a diet moderate in sugar.* The AHA encourages consumption of complex carbohydrates in the form of grains, vegetables, and legumes. Sugar intake has not been directly related to risk for cardiovascular disease, but diets high in refined carbohydrates are often high in calories and low in complex carbohydrates, fiber, and essential vitamins and minerals (American Heart Association Dietary Guidelines, Vol. 94, No. 7, 1996).

**DAIRY PRODUCTS.** Unknown to early man, fat-free dairy products are acceptable in both Katahn and Montignac diets with hard cheeses included in the Montignac protein/lipid meals.

Human breast milk was of course a Paleolithic necessity, but today's adults become lactose intolerant. (Only the northern European population has evolved or retained the ability to digest milk.) Yogurt is fermented to remove lactose which will permit all to digest it.

> *Margarine itself is cholesterol free, but that doesn't matter; it raises your cholesterol levels. Even worse, because it's high in trans-fatty acids, margarine itself is a potent enemy that will drive you out of the Zone* (Sears, 1995, p. 124).

**PREPARED FOODS.** Eliminate ersatz foods. Why retain the sweet tooth by using sugar substitutes? Simply eliminate foods and drinks that are sweetened. Eating olestrol-fried potato chips is ludicrous when one should eliminate the high glycemic potato and excess salt anyway. Forget the ice cream substitutes which provide so much sugar. Get out of the habit of canned or frozen foods (which will eliminate label analysis). Eat fresh vegetables and fruit.

> *Concentrate your grocery shopping in the outer aisles. Foods in the inner aisles are designed to have a long shelf life, and sugar is one of the commonest preservatives for this purpose. Shop the outer aisles—the produce, meat, dairy, and bulk food sections—and take some of the guesswork out of what to buy.* (Gittelman, 1996, p. 19).

**BEVERAGES**. Caffeine, sugar, and alcoholic drinks are not recommended in either diet. The Frenchman, Montignac, introduces red wine in his maintenance diet. Amazingly, the average American ingests up to 7 to 10 percent of total calories from alcohol which is devoid of nutritional value.

This chapter has been an overview of how today's age of agriculture foods relate to the Stone Age. For detailed information on both generic foods, brand names, even the fast-food chain's sandwiches and fries, read Corinne Netzer's book of food counts. (Of course many others are available.)

Her book lists calories; protein, carbohydrates, and total fat in grams; cholesterol, sodium, and fiber in milligrams. It is instructive to prepare a check list of generic items such as meats, fish, dairy products, starches, vegetables, fruits, plus your favorite "fast" foods. This is your personal guideline for any diet. It will tell you where you've been and where you are going.

Netzer's book is two inches thick in paperback and 770 pages. I still have my little *Dell Purse Guide of 1965*, carbohydrate gram counter, 64 pages, and my still smaller *Pocket Guide for Calorie Counters* (22nd printing, May 1948, 48 pages). Contrasting these little books of yesteryear to that 770 page book permits an observation. We have multiplied the book size some sixteen-fold in two generations due to tremendous growth in knowledge, but have increased obesity and cardiovascular problems proportionally. The next chapter on the Zone gives Barry Sears' account of why America has fattened—pasta, pasta, pasta, and other refined grains.

Thankfully, the trend lines of cardiovascular diseases are now moving downward but are still way up from two generations ago. In subsequent chapters, we will present the new nutrition of Linus Pauling, where he shows a direct relationship between the increased production of vitamin C and the decrease of heart and blood problems. Chapter Ten presents the aerobics of Dr. Kenneth Cooper. Although only about 25 percent of people exercise faithfully, this too has decreased the epidemic of circulatory problems.

But the most important long range factor of all is the Zone Diet—adequate protein, minimal fat, healthy, fibrous carbohydrate, full of vitamins and minerals, and the elimination of the starch deluge. So read on.

# 5

# BARRY SEARS: THE ZONE

*The Zone, A Dietary Road Map*
Barry Sears, Ph.D. & William Lawren (Regan Books, 1995)
Excerpts reprinted by permission of HarperCollins Publishers, Inc.
Copyright 1995 by Barry Sears and William Lawren
*Mastering the Zone*
Barry Sears, Ph.D. (Regan Books, 1997)
*Zone Perfect Meals in Minutes*
Barry Sears, Ph.D. (Regan Books, 1997)

Barry Sears starts *The Zone*, "A Sword of Damocles hangs over my head." At age 50 he lives with genes that caused five forbearers to succumb to heart attacks before age 54. He recounts how he has lived and worked during his productive life to understand the digestion and utilization of food to beat these odds. I believe he has succeeded. There have been no long range population studies of the Zone diet, but you will find the case histories presented exhilarating. The Zone diet works for me; it brought me below 200 pounds for the first time since age 17 in 1942 and, I'll tell you, that is like finding the Holy Grail.

"The effect of diet (particularly the protein-to-carbohydrate ratio of the meals you eat) on the metabolic fate of omega 6 fatty acids determines whether or not you will ever enter the Zone" (Sears, 1995, p. 121). Make no mistake. This is not just another diet book based on empirical or anecdotal musings. Barry Sears is a scientist. **He is the first human on this earth who has ever explained the biochemical reactions of nutrition to create a diet that will resolve the twin bugaboos of our era,** *obesity and cholesterol.*

Insulin and glucagon are hormones that control blood sugar, and are in turn controlled by eicosanoids, whose discovery won the 1982 Nobel Prize for Medicine. But little more has been published about them—until Barry Sears put it all together.

> *Eicosanoids are the most powerful biological agents known to man. Control eicosanoids and you'll open the door to the Zone* (Sears, 1995, p. 32).

He has found the mix of macronutrients—fat, carbohydrate, and protein—that will produce good eicosanoids. A bad mix—too many high glycemic starches or too much saturated fat are prime examples—will produce bad eicosanoids. The catch word "Zone" denotes that time period when we have the proper mix. Be certain, being in the Zone creates a feeling of exuberant health. Is it euphoria? Awareness? Power? Up and at 'em? And all the while, fat, detestable fat, is consumed. It works!

Euphoria aside, Barry Sears has put to rout the body's ability to defeat the laws of thermodynamics when subjected to a fat gram or a calorie counting regimen. You are not hungry when in the Zone. You are free of the yearning to drink coffee, eat a doughnut or a Snickers, have 8.5

teaspoons of sugar coke, have a martini at 5:00 pm or a smoke. The Zone evens out the level of blood sugar. It makes you a superior being.

> *You fatten cattle by feeding them lots and lots of low-fat grain. How do you fatten humans? Same way: you feed them lots and lots of low-fat grain. So if you've been eating more pasta and bread (both made from grain) than ever before, and you're still gaining weight, think about those grain-fed cattle the next time you sit down to a big plate of pasta* (Sears, 1995, p. 9).

It's amazing to compare Barry Sears with Martin Katahn.

Katahn: *Only fat makes you fat.*

Sears: *Eating fat does not make you fat.*

Katahn: *Eat, eat, carbohydrates.*

Sears: *It's your body's response to excess carbohydrates that makes you fat. You have to eat fat to lose fat!*

Sears points to the great carbohydrate experiment of the past fifteen years. Result: a 32% increase in obese Americans between 1960 and 1980. And the National Institute of Health revealed that the average weight of young Americans increased ten pounds between 1988 and 1995. The paradox: people are eating less fat but getting fatter.

Sears cites research at Stanford University in 1987 that showed wide variation in people's genetic insulin response. There are some lucky people, about 25%, who do well on a carbohydrate diet since their insulin levels are always low. But another 25% are just the opposite, and

50% are in between. Seventy-five percent of the population can profit from Sears' diet. Can you?

> *Until a decade ago, glucose was believed to be the major fuel for energy. This proved to be untrue, despite the fact that glucose is oxidized readily and even preferentially when the supply is abundant. Quantitatively, fat in the form of free fatty acids is used much more extensively. As the concentration of free fatty acids in the blood increases, the oxidation of sugar diminishes, inhibiting the use of sugar by all other tissues. Under most circumstances, fat is the major fuel for energy requirements.*
>
> *If we consider that a high concentration of free fatty acids diminishes the oxidation of sugar and that the obese person constantly has a very high concentration of these acids, we realize that he is continuously using fat for most of his metabolic functions whether or not he is eating* (Gordon, 1969, p.96).

Carbohydrates are the reason most of us are fat. Only 60 to 90 grams of carbohydrates can be stored as glycogen in the liver, about two cups of cooked pasta! The excess ends up as fat. And then the increased insulin levels make it almost impossible to use stored body fat. Sears discusses how the glycemic index of carbohydrates relates to the speed of insulin response. He advises an easily remembered rating of carbohydrates; "Virtually all fruits (except bananas and dried fruit) and virtually all fiber-rich vegetables (except carrots and corn) are low glycemic carbohydrates. Virtually all grains, starches, and pasta are high glycemic carbohydrates" (Sears, 1995, p. 18). The food pyramid diet, eating high glycemic carbohydrates, keeps us fat!

Proteins are the basis of all life, making up about one-half of our body weight. There are twenty amino acids, the building blocks of body protein, and nine of these—the essential amino acids—must be supplied by the food we eat.

> *An excess consumption of carbohydrates is known to increase the body's production of lipogenic or fat storing enzymes, such as lipoprotein lipase. The overfeeding of carbohydrates for long periods of time increases the body's ability to store calories as fat. Sugars are especially implicated in this process* (Clouatre, 1993, p. 106).
>
> *The amount of carbohydrates eaten should be kept down to the amount that permits the ingested fat to be burned rather than deposited in the body.* —Linus Pauling (1986, p. 31)

Body fat is the primary source of energy, and daily fat ingestion is the only source of the essential fatty acids that are the building blocks of life. The controlling factor in the release of fat is the balance of eicosanoids.

When in the Zone, your body is making more "good" eicosanoids than "bad," and fat can be released faster. When out of the Zone, fat release slows. This is the touchstone of the Zone diet. Body fat is reduced, not muscle or water, and the Zone is the quantified diet plan that will accomplish this.

Barry Sears shows us how to determine body fat percentage, using charts to personalize protein requirements based on your activity and your body's non-fat weight. The complete eating pattern thus is based on individual protein daily need. Carbohydrate is set at 4-parts for each 3-parts of protein. Fat in calories equals protein calories. Total diet: 30-40-30, protein-carbohydrate-fat, percentage.

Thus each person using the Zone "block" system arrives at his or her total calorie intake. This is divided into three meals of equal size and one or two snacks. Snacks should be limited to 100 calories. Meals should not be greater than 500 calories. Thus, larger people may need more meals than three each day. It is vital to ingest the same proportion of macronutrients at each meal or snack. This will access the stored fat!

Detractors of the Zone diet inveigh against the 30-40-30 percent relationship between macronutrients, calling it a "high-fat, high-protein" diet. They could not be more wrong. They have certainly not studied the diet. The crux of the Zone diet is one's individual protein needs. A voluminous bibliography of background authority for this and all other conclusions is presented on the Internet <http://www.eicotech.com>.

TABLE 8
Recommended Protein and Fat Grams
for Various Diets

| DIET (MEN) | PROTEIN (gms) | FAT (gms) |
|---|---|---|
| Consumer Reports 1992 Consensus - 2250 calories | 65 (average) | 62 |
| Adelle Davis - 1954 | 70 (average) | — |
| Dietary Goal - Senate Select Committee on Nutrition - 2500 calories | 75 (average) | 83 |
| Roy Walford, *The 120 Year Diet* | 60-90 | 30-45 |
| Martin Katahn, *The T-Factor Diet* | common levels | 30-60 |
| Cooper Clinic "*Real Life Average*" - 2050 calories | 95 | 86 |
| Barry Sears, *The Zone* | 50-110 | 27-42 |

Consider the first three items in Table 8, labeled "average." (The *Consumer Reports* 65 grams is actually overall, including women and men.) An "average" male according to nutritionists weighs 154 lbs. with 23 percent body fat. According to the Zone tables, this average male, *if inactive* would require 59 grams protein. If we include women, the average would become about 54 grams. And again, according to the National Academy of Science, "This [daily protein quantity] amounts to 56 grams for the average man and 46 for the average woman" (Walford, 1986, p. 206). Enough said?!

Just as Barry Sears says, the Zone is adequate protein and low fat! Let's expand the comparison to the Cooper Clinic study of July 1994 where 2,951 men were analyzed in five fitness categories along with their eating patterns. We extract these data by averaging the center three of five categories, removing the least and most fit. *(See Table 9.)*

### TABLE 9
### Comparison of Zone Reducing Diet and Real Life Diet

|  | Cooper Clinic *Real Life* | | Barry Sears *Light to moderate activity* | | | |
|---|---|---|---|---|---|---|
|  | | | 154-lb. Man | | 200-lb. Man | |
|  | (Cal.) | (Gm.) | (Cal.) | (Gm.) | (Cal.) | (Gm.) |
| Protein | 380 | 95 | 308 | 77 | 416 | 104 |
| Carbohydrate | 895 | 224 | 396 | 99 | 536 | 134 |
| Fat - unsaturated | 570 | 57 | 149 | 16.5 | 198 | 22 |
| Fat - saturated | 265 | 29 | 149 | 16.5 | 198 | 22 |
| **Calorie Totals** | **2050** | | **1002** | | **1348** | |

Thus the Zone diet for myself, at 200 pounds, is 702 calories less than the Cooper *Real Life* diet average, yet entirely adequate in protein, fats, and low glycemic carbohydrates, fibers, and minerals. Any other comparable diet deficit that I have undergone has been "grit your teeth." Obviously, I'm burning just as many calories, but the deficit is made up by fat stores. Barry Sears has actually made diet thermodynamics a mathematical certainty. You feel great and finally in control.

The Zone diet is remarkably low in fat and most remarkably low in calories. It is actually lower in fat than the Katahn *Low-fat* diet and slightly lower than the Walford, *120-Year* diet and much lower than *Real Life*. You eliminate the empty calories of pasta, pasta, pasta and access body fat for energy.

Figure 5 graphically portrays the Zone and the crucial role played by the protein-to-carbohydrate ratio.

**FIGURE 5**
**Pictorial Portrayal of the Zone**

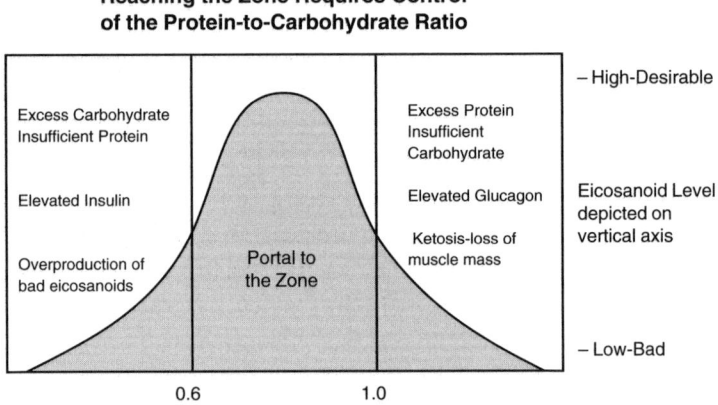

Adapted from Sears, 1995, pp. 29, 66.

The Zone is mathematically determined but covers a comfortably wide range. If the ideal is a ratio of 0.75 between protein and carbohydrate, the range that keeps us in the Zone is 0.60 to 1.0. Sears provides food selections and ways to judge quantities, so everyone can build a diet around favorite or at least reasonable foods. The building of a routine is not onerous. Sears even provides an 800 number for questions. He puts his money where his mouth is.

The fat reducing qualities of the Zone, while certainly not incidental, are actually secondary to the fact that the Zone may be a panacea for many of the diseases of civilization, those maladies that are treated but scarcely ever cured. Barry Sears is the ultimate practitioner of orthomolecular medicine, as defined by Linus Pauling later in this book (Chapter Eight).

He has perceived the elegant unity that links disease states to diet, just as Hans Selye (Chapter Nine) perceived the unity of wide ranging stresses producing the same bodily breakdowns. We can control stress with diversion; we can control diverse disease states with the Zone diet:

- **Heart disease**. Hyper- (too much) insulin production is the risk factor, according to Barry Sears, that best predicts heart attacks. This is brought on by low-fat, high carbohydrate diets, which produce bad eicosanoids.
- **High blood pressure**. Bad eicosanoids cause blood vessels to narrow and promote blood platelet clumping.
- **Obesity and Type II Diabetes**. Losing body fat has such a dramatic impact on reducing blood pressure, high cholesterol, and type II diabetes.
- **Smoking, drinking, caffeine**. Your urge for addictive dietary or sensory stimulants will disappear as you actually produce good prostaglandin (an eicosanoid) and keep blood sugar on an even keel.
- **Arterial blockage, atherosclerosis**. All promoted by bad eicosanoids.

- **Cancer.** More and more research shows the role of bad eicosanoids. The reader is urged—nay, begged—to study this chapter in the *Zone*.
- **Auto-immune diseases, arthritis.** The overproduction of bad eicosanoids causes the body to attack itself.
- **Cholesterol**

> *So let's say you're eating one of those trendy, recommended diets that's low in cholesterol and high in carbohydrate. If you're genetically predisposed to have an elevated insulin response to carbohydrates, then you're doing everything in your power to increase the body's production of cholesterol—even though there's almost no cholesterol in your diet.*
>
> *No wonder that dietary intervention to reduce cholesterol rarely seems to work. That's because no diet other than a Zone-favorable diet addresses what's really controlling your cholesterol levels: eicosanoids* (Sears, 1995, p. 144).

And on and on,
- **Chronic fatigue,**
- **Central nervous system disorder,**
- **Alcoholism,**
- **Chronic pain,**
- **Skin disorders.**

And finally,
- **Life extension.**

Roy Walford wrote *The 120-Year Diet* (1986) around the theme of calorie restricting diets increasing life spans. This is well proven in animal studies. Walford discusses glycemic index, but his diet, based on 20% protein and 20% fat, is a tough one for the 75% of us with Paleolithic genes, and it drives you out of the Zone.

The Zone diet is calorie restricting, but it is not doomed to failure because of over-ingestion of carbohydrates. You can live your whole life in the Zone, pleasantly, happily, energetically, and it may well be a far longer life! You are not hungry in the Zone.

These wellness conclusions result from Sears' great expertise in studying the body's responses to hormones produced by food and to his knowledge of the same responses produced by specific drugs. Many interesting case histories resulted from individuals who started the Zone diet to lose fat, but who reported that long established medical conditions also melted away!

Here are Barry Sears' conclusions:
- Despite eating less fat, Americans are fatter than ever. Why? Because fat does not make you fat; insulin does. There are two ways to increase insulin—eat too much food at any one meal, or eat too many carbohydrates.
- Eating fat doesn't make you fat, as long as it's the right type of fat. Mono-unsaturated fat has no effect on insulin. If you're eating too many carbohydrates, adding any type of fat is a real prescription for rapid fat gain.
- Athletes perform better on a high-fat diet than on a high carbohydrate diet.
- Exercise alone will rarely overcome the negative effects of a high-carbohydrate diet.
- For cardiovascular patients, a high-carbohydrate diet may be hazardous to their health.
- Food may be the most powerful drug you will ever take. Hormones are hundreds of times stronger than drugs.
- The new dietary recommendations of the U.S. Government nutrition experts and medical experts are dead wrong. If the base of the Pyramid diet were

simply thrown away, you'd be left with a Zone-favorable diet.
- The quality of your life is controlled by the Zone. In the Zone, you can modify the expression of your genetic destiny, ultimately reaching your full genetic potential.
- Don't be misled by the apparent simplicity of this dietary program to reach the Zone. A Zone-favorable diet, if properly followed, produces fundamental changes at the hormone level that everyone can achieve (Sears, 1995, p. 207-09).

> *In other words, once the medical establishment finally understands the potential of diet to alter eicosanoids, that should revolutionize the current practice of medicine* (Sears, 1995, p. 21).

Two generations ago, Adelle Davis in her wonderful book, *Let's Eat Right To Keep Fit*, described the diet of one of her acquaintances. He was in ebullient health, more energetic and mentally alert than he'd been in years. His diet: protein, fat, and carbohydrates at every meal and particularly a good breakfast. He was in the Zone!

Her book glorifies proper nutrition. To read the 31 chapter titles is to obtain a short course in health. We discuss three of them which have been quantified by Sears.

- *Breakfast Gets The Day's Work Done* (Davis, 1970, p. 20).
- *The Stuff You're Made Of* (Davis, 1970, p. 29). Protein at each meal creates the zest and level of efficiency in the hours until next eating. And the corollary is fat.

She even commits the apostasy of stating that a cause of overweight can be too little fat—a fact now repeated by Sears. Of course, much discussion by each expert gives us their reasoning and limitations. *You need your health and your zest and your aliveness to burn calories and create a shapely body.*
- *Can We Prevent Being Deluged* (Davis, 1970, p. 50). Sugar and its corollary, starch. There is little point in a comment here. I did certainly enjoy her statements on school lunch programs, which keep newly appearing paraphrased in the media, but with little avail. If you will read her comments on the refining of foods, particularly the milling of grain, you will almost certainly "shop the outer aisles!"

While contemplating the state of our high glycemic, fatty, current dining, it is pitiable now to see how right Adelle Davis was forty years ago.

But eating beliefs die hard. At least two reports from prestigious institutions, widely quoted in publications, roundly castigate Barry Sears and the Zone. These are the May 1996 Tufts University Diet and Health Letter and the January 1997 Harvard Health Letter. The reader is urged to study these criticisms and to study critically the Zone. Discuss them with your medical advisors, have a blood profile, conclude whether you could or should try the Zone plan for a time period of weight loss. By all means do it if medical advice permits, then obtain a second blood profile.

I have done this and have never, in 29 years of blood profiles—the last 24 at the Cooper Clinic in Dallas—had higher HDL cholesterol and lower HDL to total cholesterol ratio, than my test 7/29/97. These results were 67 and 2.6 respectively (improved from April 1996 at 54 and

3.0) after six months in the Zone (80% of the time) and a 13-pound weight loss. LDL remained the same, HDL increased 13 points, and triglycerides were down 11% to 40.

The nubs of criticism (in parentheses):

- *(The Zone recommends protein at an unhealthy high level.)* The best data this writer obtained is presented in this chapter. The Zone is protein adequate.
- *(The Zone causes ketosis.)* It does not. It is designed not to. (Ketosis is described in Chapter Three.)
- *(The Zone is much too low in carbohydrate.)* Actually the Zone is very high in good carbohydrates, micronutrients, vitamins, minerals and fibers. Much more than the Pyramid Diet.
- *(The Zone is ridiculously low in calories.)* Some sort of a *non sequitur*. Actually the Zone provides all the protein, fat and low glycemic nutrients your body requires. The calorie deficit is made up from body fat stores.
- *(The Zone simply cannot reduce hunger because it is so low in calories, thus is a difficult diet, and besides requires slavish counting.)* All incorrect. Your body does not perceive a calorie deficit because there isn't one. Not with the Zone access to body fat, which is its miracle. You are only hungry at meal time in the Zone. The range of nutrients is comfortably high allowing for easy approximations. For example, for every 100 calories of protein, a range of 100 to 150 calories of carbohydrates will keep you in the Zone. And meat/fish quantity is approximated by the palm of your hand. Stay away from starches and sugar, and the proportions just about take care of themselves.
- *(The Zone cannot help medical conditions.)* Those good blood profiles from the Zone truly should help alleviate the diseases of civilization, and fortunately

some doctors agree. I received my copy of the Zone book from a friend who has been given this diet by her oncologist. Another friend with adult onset diabetes has been given the Zone diet by her doctor.

Well, reader, for myself I want to drop another 12 pounds and then decide if I want to gormandize a bit. As Barry Sears says, if you fall out of the Zone, all it takes is to start again at the next meal.

In Chapter Four we referred to the Cooper Clinic Tip Sheet, "Optimal Nutrition" (see Appendix Two), as well as the book, *The Balancing Act, Nutrition and Weight Guide* by Georgia G. Kostas, Director of Nutrition at the Cooper Clinic. These are excellent statements on the current establishment Pyramid diet and should be part of everyone's lexicon. My Zone diet varies in the following fashions, otherwise it is right on!

- My three daily meals are of equal caloric amounts and nutrient distribution. I wake up to the day actually hungry, not still bloated up with 40% of yesterday's calories.
- I omit the refined starches and most root vegetables. These are misnamed "complex carbohydrates," but I term them "empty" carbohydrate because the newest nutritional science proves what Adelle Davis stated 44 years ago—that they add to the sugar deluge. We now know that many refined starches are higher in glycemic value than white sugar. Barry Sears says to substitute water for the starches in the Pyramid diet and you have a better diet. I substitute literally buckets full of green vegetables high in "complex" micronutrients and vitamins. (A little hyperbole, but you do not lack for food quantity in the Zone.)

- The Tip Sheet shows 10% to 20% protein, and I will assume that the diet allows 2,400 daily calories. This is about 240 to 480 calories of protein or 60 to 120 grams. I eat about 90 grams, right in the middle. The point here is how do Harvard and Tufts get away with terming the Zone diet high protein and inveighing against it? Do they also criticize the Pyramid diet?
- The Tip Sheet shows 20 to 30% fat, again assuming 2,400 calories, 480 to 720 calories of fat. This becomes about 53 to 80 grams fat. My fat intake in the Zone is 21 added unsaturated fat grams over and above another 21 grams assumed to be entrained in the protein items eaten. The Zone reducing diet is actually a low-fat diet, lower than the American Heart Association guidelines.

*Outdoor* magazine has a September, 1997 article entitled "Dr. Feelbetter" by Paul Keegan detailing much of the controversy. He bemoans that the dispute could be resolved through reason and rigorous scientific experimentation, and so it could. But *deja vu*, it took thirty years before Linus Pauling was vindicated. It has taken twenty years before homocysteine (Chapter Four) saw the light of day.

And finally what did that 13-pound weight loss do for body fat? At the Cooper Clinic in Dallas 7/29/97, my weight was 203 lbs. After six months in the Zone, I had cut approximately 2 inches from my waist requiring trousers to be taken in and a new set of walking shorts, and even more upper abdominal fat loss. I am buttoning 15-year-old sports jackets. Percent body fat via the pinch method was 21.7% on 7/29/97 compared to 26.3% on 7/14/94, my last such determination. At a 1994 weight of 214 lbs., this represents a 4.6% loss, which multiplied by 214 lbs. indicates approximately a 10 lb. loss. Very close to the actual 11 lb. loss and ostensibly a fat loss.

But ambiguity rears its ugly head. Percent body fat figured by the underwater weighing method remained exactly the same, which could indicate a loss of LBM (lean body mass). Using the Zone tables of percent body fat, I can verify that my weight loss is fat loss, but the LBM, so determined, is yet a third figure. No matter, my sport jackets still fit the way they are supposed to, but where does that leave exact wisdom for you, the reader.

Obviously, tests conducted under research study guidelines should be made. Meanwhile, we must make considered choices while we are still on this earth. What Paul Keegan's article does not state, much less the Harvard and Tufts critiques, is that the Zone diet makes you feel A-OK. *The calorie counting, pasta-pasta-pasta diets fail because you do not stabilize blood sugar.*

So how is life in the Zone? Approaching 73, I'm super-energized all day. Thirty-five years ago after my toast and jam (but no butter) breakfast following the previous evening's big dinner, I would fight mental fatigue until the doughnut break. Have you noticed yourself hungry two hours after a big pasta or rice meal? Do you yearn for petty addictions such as snacks, colas, or cocktails even though logic tells you you've had plenty of calories? The Zone resolves these blahs, the mood swings, and the high-lows.

I have tried to poke a hole into the Zone balloon. I have yet to read any scholarly, critical analysis of the Zone. I've tried to emphasize key points and to be a critic. I've even added the Zone diet precepts into the recommended Pyramid diet and can't see any nutrients missing except high caloric density starch—and good riddance. And I'm convinced that the diseases of civilization will be immeasurably reduced by it. Let us continue our wellness quest with further corroboration.

# 6

# THE PROMISED LAND

**The Diet and Health Benefits of HCA**
Dallas Clouatre & Michael Rosenbaum (Keats Publishing, 1994)
**Getting Lean with Anti-fat Nutrients**
Dallas Clouatre (Pax Publishing, 1996)

For yo-yo diet afficionados, the Zone diet truly works. And for those who are able to count calories, perhaps a safe, effective, weight-loss "silver bullet" does exist. HCA (hydroxycitric acid) is extracted from the dried rind of the exotic fruit from the East Indian Garcinea Gambogia tree. It not only gives you more energy while lessening the appetite, but also helps prevent the carbohydrates you consume in starches, fruits, vegetables, and sugars from being converted into fat. HCA is the first natural weight loss compound that accomplishes this without adversely affecting the central nervous system and causing side effects such as anxiety or jitters.

The following are some observations made by Clouatre and Rosenbaum about HCA (1994, p. 6):

- **HCA reduces** the rate of conversion of dietary carbohydrate calories to fat, i.e., it inhibits lipogenesis.
- **The production of low density lipoprotein (LDL) and triglycerides**—HCA may lower the production of both cholesterol and fatty acids as a result of its effects upon metabolism.
- **Energy levels and glycogen storage**—experimental evidence shows that HCA increases the production of glycogen in the liver (and probably in peripheral tissues), which promises greater and more sustained energy for those with glycogen storage problems.
- **Appetite control**—preclinical and clinical evidence indicate that HCA suppresses appetite and thereby reduces food intake, although exact dosage levels remain to be established.
- **Thermogenesis**—some authors speculate that HCA may increase the body's production of heat, burning calories in response to food consumption by activating the process of thermogenesis.

The Bronson (800/235-3200) HCA comes complete with a calorie counting diet. The value of HCA is that it apparently works as an appetite suppressant. I can report that in 1996 I took HCA for a period of 8 months—three 250mg capsules daily before meals. My weight remained constant with an actual four-pound loss without dieting during this period that included considerable traveling. HCA removes desire for snacking or eating between meals.

July 8, 1996, the *Milwaukee Journal Sentinel* reported (bylined by Julie Sevrens) that the FDA has approved the first anti-obesity drug in 22 years, Redux. A few side effects were noted: pulmonary hypertension, diarrhea, drowsiness, dry mouth, and headaches. A spokesperson was quoted as saying that "diets don't work; we need to alter the satiety centers in the brain."

Sept. 16, 1997, the *Milwaukee Journal Sentinel* reported (bylined by Marlene Cimons) that the FDA had requested removal from the market of two diet drugs, Redux and Pondimin, as 92 out of 291 patients using the drugs had damaged heart valves.

And again, the *Milwaukee Journal Sentinel* ran a full page ad on September 16, 1996 extolling the new Absorb-A11 Super Formula fat blocker, a 60-day supply for $89.95. This formula does contain HCA, chromium picolinate, and several other more esoteric ingredients. You will lose weight while harmful cholesterol and triglycerides are blocked from your system. No side effects were noted.

Dallas Clouatre's book, *Getting Lean with Anti-Fat Nutrients*, provides details on 17 fat controlling nutrients. Many of these are vitamins and antioxidants that we should take in any case. **But of course our goal is to adopt a lifelong eating pattern that will please our gastronomy and our healthy physique without developing a dependency on diet "aids."**

> *Rather, it (food) is a potent drug that you'll take at least three times a day for the rest of your life. Once food is broken down into its basic components (glucose, amino acids, and fatty acids) and sent into the bloodstream, it has a more powerful impact on your body—and your health—than any drug your doctor could ever prescribe* (Sears, 1995, p. 77).

A fine analysis of diet information appears in the last three chapters of Clouatre's book. These chapters, "Food Factors," "The End of Dieting," and "The Cholesterol Controversy," are jewels of brevity. Everyone is urged to study them. We will attempt to provide commentary on those items that clarify the themes of *Starch Madness*. Dallas Clouatre appears to be one of those experts who has arrived at a Paleolithic diet without calling it such. He provides food couplings for weight loss that corroborate the Montignac maintenance diet.

**EXAMPLE MENUS**
from Clouatre that corroborate Montignac

**Protein-based Breakfast:** Cheese omelet, Spanish tomatoes and bell peppers, beverage

**Carbohydrate-based Lunch:** Baked potato, peas and pearl onions in curry sauce, corn and red bell peppers, ½ cup raspberries, beverage.

**Protein-based Dinner:** Chicken breast, vegetable soup, sautéed pea pods with mushrooms, asparagus, salad (walnut oil and vinegar), sugar-free sherbet, beverage.

Key #1: Avoid fat/simple carbohydrate combinations. Avoid all sugars. Eat no more than two servings of fruit a day and drink no fruit juices. Limit protein/carbohydrate combinations.

Key #2: Couple proteins with vegetables. Trim the visible fats from meats, but do not attempt to make protein meals "fat-free." You can eat unlimited amounts of non-starchy (primarily green) vegetables and limited amounts of starchy vegetables at protein-containing meals.

Key #3: Couple complex carbohydrates /starches with vegetables. Avoid fats and limit protein (less than ¼ cup) at carbohydrate containing meals. Small amounts (¼ cup) of all nuts (raw) except peanuts can be eaten.

Annotated from *Anti-Fat Nutrients* by Dallas Clouatre, Ph.D. Copyright 1993 by Dallas Clouatre. Published by Pax Publishing, San Francisco, CA 94122. Reprinted by permission.

All of this is now familiar. *"The dieter's dilemma is that, with low-calorie diets, you must cut calories to lose weight. Yet cutting calories itself slows the calorie burning process"* (Clouatre, 1990, p. 80). Weight loss is easy; fat loss is not. The manifesto: Down with sugar and up with metabolism inducing exercise!

Plan on walking 30 minutes each day. This is best either before or just after breakfast; it will turn on your fat burning powers. Fibrous green vegetables will slow down digestion. Never skip breakfast. Eat the evening meal at least three hours before bedtime. Avoid caffeine which can upset sleep. Eating late close to bedtime makes the food available for fat after the body has begun to slow down for sleep. Then, glycogen stores being sated, one may not eat breakfast. Breakfast signals the body that it is free to expend energy. More energy is consumed after exercise because the metabolic rate is raised, then burned during the exercise.

On a reducing diet with an absence of carbohydrates, the body will break down fat, and to a lesser degree will break down protein. Thus carbohydrate and protein should be adequate—and adequate 24 hours of the day (as they are in the Zone)—to promote fat-only weight loss. This corroborates the Zone diet!

While non-obese individuals can overeat carbohydrates for periods of time, over a long time this leads to fat storage. It is also true that on mixed diets, overeating fat is more likely to lead to weight gain than overeating carbohydrates. However insulin reactions are magnified by high glycemic refined carbohydrates, and by body type!

Clouatre cites a considerable bibliography to indicate that sugar increases liver enzymes, elevating blood fat (triglycerides). He particularly indicts fructose. Remember that we learned in Chapter Four that 50 percent of sugar, sucrose, converts to fructose. Fructose elevates insulin and uric acid levels and, according to Linus Pauling, may be a precursor to cholesterol deposits. All that said, do we now give up fruit, which provides fructose? It would appear prudent to follow the 1992 *Consumer Reports* guidelines of limiting sugar to 5 percent of our diet and to include fruit "sugar," fructose, in this 5 percent. In the Zone diet, sweeteners are very much curtailed.

*(And here I note the latest fad in jams and jellies—natural sweeteners, no sugar, just concentrated fruit juice—pure fructose. Someone who had not read Linus Pauling started this one.)*

This analysis by Clouatre goes far to explain the wide disparity of the research of Katahn and the basis of the Pyramid type diets vis-à-vis Montignac and Sears. This book tries to work through the labyrinth, allowing us to select the proper aspects of all the advice for our own body type.

Is it not frightening to read in this chapter the quotation in the news article on Redux: "Diets don't work; we need to alter the satiety centers in the brain"? You can be sure that drug company research continues. In his Preface to *The Zone,* Sears recounts how his research led him to detailed knowledge of metabolism and led him to his conclusions that the most powerful "drug" was food.

In the next chapter we learn almost equally astounding truisms about an even more commonplace "nutrient"—water.

# 7

# YOUR BODY'S MANY CRIES FOR WATER

*Your Body's Many Cries for Water*
Dr. Fereydoon Batmanghelidj
(Global Health Solutions, 1992) 800/759-3999
*Chapter title and quotations reprinted with permission.*

When the human body is chronically deprived of water, its automatic defense mechanism kicks in to conserve water for vital body functions at the expense of other areas. Conditions then arise that mimic disease. Treatments attempted with over-the-counter or prescribed drugs only exacerbate the problems. "It is chronic dehydration that is the root cause of many of the diseases we confront in medicine at present" (Batmanghelidj, 1995, p. 2). Dr. Batmanghelidj, an Iranian by birth, has had a lifelong interest in the effects of water. He was educated at the University of London and now lives in Virginia.

Many of these symptoms appear to be the diseases of civilization referred to in Chapter One. Let us examine

these diseases and the role played by chronic dehydration, which may be too slight to create a "dry mouth" thirst sensation:
- Dyspeptic pain or heart burn is a thirst signal associated with chronic or severe dehydration in the human body. It should be treated by the regular intake of water. Current treatment and use of antacids and histamine blocking agents does not benefit a chronically dehydrated person whose body has resorted to crying for water.
- Colitis pain may result from lack of water as might constipation.
- Rheumatoid arthritis pain should initially be viewed as a water deficiency in the cartilage surfaces. "In a well-hydrated cartilage, the rate of friction damage is minimal" (Batmanghelidj, 1995, p. 43).
- Spinal pain may be caused by a lack of water in the discs, whose composition is 75 percent water.
- Hypertension or high blood pressure is an adaptive process to a gross water deficiency" (Batmanghelidj, 1995, p. 65). When there is a decrease in total fluid volume in the body (blood plus water) because of a water shortage, then blood circulation "gates" are closed to prevent blood volume loss which would otherwise flow into the tissues because of the water imbalance. Thus is blood pressure increased.
- Obesity may be due to an interpretation of the thirst sensation as hunger. Drinking water before eating may doubly be a panacea. It may remove the desire to overeat!
- Water retention, amazingly, may be effectively treated with plentiful water. The body need not conserve.
- Asthma and allergies are indicators that the body is producing histamine to regulate evaporative loss of

water by constricting the bronchial tubes. One wonders how many over-the-counter medications tell you to be sure to drink eight glasses of water daily.

This is not all. My goodness, I am a health enthusiast who is getting older and know that older folk may lose their thirst sensation. I so well remember my mother-in-law being treated with diuretics—just wrong!

Dehydrating agents are found in many common beverages: coffee, manufactured drinks, beers, and alcoholic concoctions. Upon awakening, the "fuzzy mouth" sensation is due to a previous evening's libations. Unfortunately, thirst may seem to be assuaged with a cola from which you get a sugar rush, or coffee which gives you a temporary nudge. You are actually depriving yourself of vital water. Drinking eight glasses of water daily can avoid dependency on coffee, beer, colas, and the like. "Alcohol, coffee, tea, and caffeine containing beverages don't count as water" (Batmanghelidj, 1995, p. 123).

> *"Water is the fourth major nutrient. ... A larger intake of water, preferably 3-liters per day is needed for the best of health." Dilute urine reduces the burden on the kidneys. There is less chance that crystals ... will form out of body fluids which can cause joint problems (gout) or kidney stones* (Pauling, 1986, p. 30).

Barry Sears feels that the ubiquitous food pyramid should be changed. The lowest tier with the 11 servings of pasta and the like should be eliminated and replaced by water.

One wonders if this writer's body, half again more hefty than his wife's, should drink the same 8 glasses of water she drinks? The indicator may be urine color which should be quite white if dilute. Dr. Kenneth Cooper's recommended water intake in cups is:

|  | ACTIVITY LEVEL | | |
|---|---|---|---|
| WEIGHT | LIGHT | MEDIUM | STRENUOUS |
| 115# | 9 | 9.5 | 10 |
| 150# | 9 | 10 | 11.5 |
| 200# | 9.5 | 11 | 13 |

From *Advanced Nutritional Theories*, Cooper, 1996, p. 331.

# 8

# THE NEW NUTRITION

*How to Live Longer and Feel Better*
Linus Pauling, Ph.D.
(W.H. Freeman & Co., 1986)
*Vitamin C and the Common Cold and the Flu*
Linus Pauling, Ph.D.
(W.H. Freeman & Co., 1970)

"*Not only will men of science have to grapple with the sciences that deal with man, but—and this is a far more difficult matter—they will have to persuade the world to listen to what they have to say.*"

These words by Bertrand Russell, cherished by Hans Selye, apply to Linus Pauling with special poignancy. Linus Pauling has given us his great testament, *How to Live Longer and Feel Better*, at least partially in answer to his detractors.

Nonagenarian, scientist, chemist, physicist, crystallographer, molecular biologist, medical researcher, and winner of *two* Nobel prizes two generations ago, Linus Pauling belongs in the pantheon of history's great minds. His great teaching was to advise us on the optimum supplementary amounts of the essential vitamins. But the old beliefs die hard. Those of us who have removed colds from our lives since his 1970 book, *Vitamin C and the Common Cold and the Flu* (read Chapter 8, *Vitamin C and Evolution*, for more Paleolithic information), shake our heads at the 1990 *Consumer Reports* mass mailing soliciting subscriptions to their health letter by espousing the very conservative view that vitamin supplements are nonessential. Now, three years after the death of Linus Pauling, we have the Anti-oxidant Revolution. In his 1986 book, only 35 of 274 pages are devoted to vitamin C, but it remains the subject most people associate with Linus Pauling.

He presents a lucid biochemical explanation of vitamin C. Our bodies cannot produce vitamin C. A reducing agent, vitamin C, together with vitamin E, protects cell membranes against damage, so that they cannot be readily entered by virus particles. Required in the body for synthesis of collagen, vitamin C is vital in connective tissue. It is known to have antibacterial action, to promote healing of wounds, broken bones, burns, and gum disease. And it is safe. No cases of kidney stone formation have been reliably reported, although adverse statements persist due to a spurious report of 20 years ago. Linus Pauling states that the only side effect is laxative action that can be used to good purpose. Vitamin C is so innocuous that we do not know what the maximum tolerable amount is. The controversy among tests for its use in combating the common cold is caused by the very small dose used in adverse tests. It works when proper amounts are used.

Pauling was conducting research into the molecular basis of mental disease at the age of 62, in 1963. He details how this led him step-by-step in the broad study of nutrition where he was astounded at the value of B vitamins. He learned of high-level vitamin C usage from Dr. Irwin

Stone and explains how his positive conclusions for increased vitamin C arose. The largest section of his book is devoted to orthomolecular medicine, defined as a way to preserve good health and to treat disease by varying the concentration in the human body of substances normally present and required for health, *thus the Anti-oxidant Revolution*. Chapters are presented on the various disease groupings.

> *Drugs are dangerous; vitamins are safe. The vitamins are foods—essential food required by human beings for life and good health. They are safe, even when used in large amounts. Side effects are infrequent and rarely serious. Also, vitamins are inexpensive compared to most drugs* (Pauling, 1986, p. 238).

Linus Pauling has concluded that the fat in food-cholesterol in the bloodstream is not the adverse cause and effect as claimed. The two pervasive afflictions of our modern era are obesity and arteriosclerosis. Two hundred years ago, our sweets intake from fruit and honey was 15 pounds annually and heart attacks were rare. During the modern era, sugar consumption has increased tenfold, with 25 percent of calories derived from it. He reports that John Yudkin of the University of London concludes that our average annual intake of 120 pounds of sugar increases risk of heart disease by a factor of six. And a 150-pound intake increases it by 15.

Linus Pauling's book discusses, on a broad scale, our state-of-the-art knowledge of all aspects of life and should be studied in that light. Unfortunately the media has overblown dissent of vitamin C into a denial of Pauling's entire work. Happily, the medical community's appreciation of him is on the upswing. In 1990, the National Cancer Institute (NCI) and National Academy of Sciences recommended increased intake of vitamin C. Large scale studies are at last underway. Also 1990 saw the NCI as host of a worldwide conference on relationships between cancer and vitamin C. NCI epidemiologist Gladys Block reviewed 47 studies, 34 of which showed that vitamin C had preventative value against cancer of the lung, stomach, colon, and on and on. Increased use of the antioxidants C, E, and beta carotene is now recommended by most medical practitioners.

**Dr. Kenneth Cooper's antioxidant recommendations:**
*We now recommend to all of our patients that they begin antioxidant therapy. The following vitamins are recommended. They may have some effect on preventing cancer, cataracts, progressive arteriosclerosis and coronary artery disease. To see positive benefits, you must consume a minimum of 1000mg of vitamin C, 400 ICU of vitamin E (in the natural or di-alpha tocopherol form) and 25,000 ICU of beta carotene per day. These are all antioxidants that interact with the free radicals which very likely are precursors of cataracts, arteriosclerosis, cancer and may even slow down aging. More recent data indicates that these antioxidants may help your immune system* (Cooper letter, 1994, to author).

In 1993, Linus Pauling's 92nd birthday marked the 20th anniversary of the Linus Pauling Institute of Science and Medicine. Its research into heart disease may be another breakthrough. Low density lipoprotein (LDL) is not deposited in atherosclerotic plaques. Lipoprotein (A), which is present in susceptible people and not to a great degree in the unaffected, becomes a surrogate for ascorbate and is deposited to strengthen blood vessels weakened by a lack of collagen and elastin.

Is heart disease an early stage of scurvy? The usual experts have been strangely silent. Pauling may be right! The proper amount of vitamin C is a must! This is one

## Treasured letter from Dr. Linus Pauling, received by author March 16, 1987.

LINUS PAULING INSTITUTE of SCIENCE and MEDICINE
440 Page Mill Road, Palo Alto, California 94306
Telephone: (415) 327-4064

16 March 1987

Mr. Richard L. Heinrich
W326 N7074 Clearwater Drive
Hartland, WI 53029

Dear Mr. Heinrich:

    I thank you for sending me a copy of the book about eating fat and growing slim, which I have read with interest.

    I think that there may be much truth in the statement that it is carbohydrate that makes people fat, not the fat in the diet.

    I thank you also for your comments on my book.

Sincerely

*Linus Pauling*

LP:dm

more reason to ingest adequate vitamin C. Who can wait for long-range epidemiological studies when vitamin C has so many life saving properties?

Linus Pauling's summary recommendations are these: "... take the optimum supplementary amount of each of the essential vitamins every day. The revolution that is taking place now liberates us from the obsession to restrict our diet, refrain from eating those foods that we like. The only limitations that I suggest are that you not eat large amounts of food and that you limit your intake of the sugar, sucrose" (Pauling, 1986, p. 274).

**Note:** The source I recommend for vitamins and food supplements is Bronson Pharmaceutical (800/235-3200 for their catalog). Its very complete listing and price list does not have the typical sales hype. As the source of Pauling's vitamin C, it is available in every conceivable formulation. The calcium ascorbate powder I use has a very neutral taste and includes the desired calcium. Ask for the AARP discount.

Another excellent source is the *Cooper Complete,* formulated by the Cooper Clinic in conjunction with experts from Harvard, Tufts, and the University of Texas to provide a daily vitamin complex (phone 888/393-2221).

Postscript: Linus Pauling died in 1994 at the age of 93. 1996 marked the prestigious joining of the Linus Pauling Institute as a research entity on the Oregon State University campus.

# 9

# TAKING STRESS IN STRIDE

*The Stress of Life*
Dr. Hans Selye (McGraw-Hill Book Co., rev. 1976)
*Personal Best*
Dr. George Sheehan (Rodale Press, 1989)

*The Stress of Life* by Dr. Hans Selye is the author's seminal treatise on the defining of and coping with stress. He says, *"This book is dedicated to those who are not afraid to enjoy the stress of a full life, nor so naïve as to think that they do so without intellectual effort."*

Dr. Selye, an Austrian, was a medical student in the 1920s in Prague when he observed that patients suffering from many specific, diagnosed causes exhibited similar non-specific responses. They looked and acted ill, had fever, coated tongues, diffuse aches, intestinal disturbances, and appetite loss. He observed that mental anguish, physical overuse, job impotence, or just overwork created the same responses. This **nonspecific response is stress**. The cause is a stressor.

In the 1930s as a researcher at McGill University (he later headed the Institute of Experimental Medicine and Surgery at Montreal), Hans Selye observed certain internal body changes: adrenal cortex enlargement, thymus gland, spleen, and lymph node changes. The ultimate example is shock. Autopsy reveals a characteristic triad of reactions: adrenocortical enlargement and increased corticoid in the blood, thymicolymphatic atrophy, and bleeding erosions in the gastrointestinal tract. **Actual quantitative biochemical measurements demonstrated that certain reactions of the body are totally nonspecific and common to all types of exposure.**

His research provided a profile of adrenocortical activity which he defines as General Adaptation Syndrome (GAS). The initial stage is the alarm reaction which creates a surge of adrenaline (corticoid activity). This is followed by the stage of resistance or adaptation where corticoid is only slightly raised. If this adaptive stage is overused, a stage of exhaustion can occur after corticoid activity peaks. Only the most severe stress leads to "shock." Most physical or mental exertions act for a limited time, and the body adapts from even a severe local stress. Dr. Selye terms this adaptive energy Local Adaptation Syndrome (LAS). Only when the whole organism is exhausted do we enter the terminal stage.

He uses exercise as an example. This produces an initial alarm reaction, warming up the muscles and cardiovascular system, followed by the stages of adaptation when we are working out in fine fettle (second wind?), but eventually exhaustion sets in. This is localized and after required rest, we recover.

Barry Sears on diet stresses:

*The final influence on GLA (gamma linolenic acid, an essential fatty acid) formation is stress. In an increasingly complex society, stress is a constant companion. It has a dramatic impact on us emotionally and physically. The body reacts to stress by producing elevated blood levels of the hormones adrenaline and cortisol. Elevated adrenaline decreases the activity of the enzyme that makes GLA, and that in turn decreases the production of good eicosanoids. Cortisol increases insulin levels, leading to an overproduction of bad eicosanoids. So stress is like a one-two punch. It does a great job of keeping you away from the Zone* (Sears, 1995, p. 124).

Dr. Batmanghelidj on dehydration stresses:

*When the body becomes dehydrated, the physiological processes that will establish are the same as coping with stress. Dehydration equals stress and once stress establishes, there is an associated mobilization of primary materials from the body stores. This process will "mop up" some of the water reserves of the body. Consequently, dehydration causes stress and stress will cause further dehydration* (Batmanghelidj, 1992, p. 52).

But, says Selye, we can and must adapt to stress to perform all the activities and face all the demands of man's lot. It is necessary to be keyed up to accomplish life's work, technically intoxicated with our own stress hormones. But it is also necessary to tone down. No one part of the body must be disproportionately overworked for a long period of time. **Systematic stress is the great equalizer.** Any intense reaction in one part can influence and equalize biological activities in others.

Selye sets up a stress quotient; local stress in any part divided by total stress in the body. **Diversion is needed,** if there is disproportionate stress in one area. And **rest is required,** if there is too much stress in the body as a whole. A workout is a diversion from mental activity, as are dancing, music, and reading. Physical activity creates a general tiredness that replenishes the body as a whole.

The most diverse aggressions can be met with the same adaptive defense mechanisms.

A simplified way to understand why stress adaptation works, and why a "good" stress such as exercise can lessen a "bad" stress such as a work or mental problem, is that stresses are not additive in an arithmetic sense. A second or third stress drains off the bad results from the single stress **if there is a deviation**. This is particularly true in general exercise stress that primes the body for rest. Mental or work stresses fall to a secondary position as exercise uses up the corticoids produced by the "bad" stress.

**Mental disposition can be dictated by appearance. Looking fit equates to feeling fit; discipline, to morale. Being in shape lessens stress.**

Self-observable signs of stress are manifold: irritability, excitation, dryness of throat, fatigue, nervous laughter or speech, sweating, frequency of urination, queasiness, headache, muscle spasm, appetite, smoking, drugs, insomnia, and ultimately, illness or neurotic behavior. The poet, Christina Rossetti, says it best, *"Who has seen the wind, neither I nor you, but when the leaves hang trembling, the wind is passing through."*

> *Sleep can result from the stress of the day, or stress can keep you awake. A work load should be planned so that daily segments can be completed, providing satisfaction. Work cares should be left at work. Mental activity that leads to a solution creates sleep but contemplating self-maintaining problems creates insomnia* (paraphrased from the teachings of Hans Selye).

Serious illness can result from sustained, long term stress. Hans Selye has researched the role of the adrenals in the spontaneous renal and cardiovascular diseases of man, inflammation diseases, digestive diseases, nervous and mental diseases, and ultimate aging. There is no question, says Selye, that all are interrelated to stress.

Dr. George Sheehan in *Runner's World* (Nov. 1978) quotes Nietzsche, "*What does not destroy me makes me strong.*"

Sheehan adds, "*Stress makes us fit, ready of mind, people of virtue and courage. Stress is what makes us complete. Through it we advance, grow, stay alive.*"

Hans Selye proved from physiological measurements and post mortems that exercise reduces stress. It fell to Dr. Kenneth Cooper, in 1968, to quantify its palliative effect.

---

Dr. George Sheehan on stress diversion and spectators in 1975 Runner's World article "From the Moment You Become a Spectator Everything is Downhill."

"*The weakest among us can become some kind of an athlete, but only the strongest can survive as spectators. Only the hardiest can withstand the perils of inertia, inactivity and immobilization. Only the most resilient can cope with the squandering of time, the deterioration of fitness, the loss of creativity, the frustration of emotions and the dulling of moral sense that can afflict the dedicated spectator ... The seated spectator is not a thinker, he is a knower. Unlike the athlete who is still seeking his own experience, who leaves himself open to truth, the spectator has closed the ring ... he is watching people who have everything he wants and cannot get. They are having all the fun: the fun of playing, the fun of winning, even the fun of losing. They are having the physical exhaustion which is the quickest way to fraternity and equality, the exhaustion which permits you to be not only a good winner but a good loser. Because the spectator cannot experience what the athlete is experiencing, the fan is seldom a good loser. The emphasis on winning is therefore much more of a problem for the spectator than the athlete.*"

# 10
# AND THE WORD WAS AEROBICS*

**Aerobics**
Maj. Kenneth Cooper (M. Evans & Co., 1968)
**The New Aerobics**
Dr. Kenneth Cooper (M. Evans & Co., 1970)
**The Aerobics Program for Total Well-Being**
Dr. Kenneth H. Cooper (M. Evans & Co., 1982)
Teachings and quotations are reprinted with honor by permission from Kenneth H. Cooper, M.D. M.P.H., president and founder, The Cooper Clinic, Dallas, Texas

Dr. Kenneth Cooper concluded early on that rhythmic exercise must be a panacea for all man's ills. His life's work has served to provide incontrovertible proof that "aerobics," the word he coined to describe this form of exercise, would be beneficial to mankind. He has accomplished this. The book is *Aerobics* and its several sequels.

---

*Title of *Runner's World* article by John Brant, May 1987.

His initial effort was to define fitness and to quantify the conditioned person. He measured the volume of air (oxygen uptake) consumed at varying work levels, correlating this into a point system. First described in his revolutionary 1968 *Readers Digest* article, "How to Feel Fit at Any Age," *aerobics,* defined as "repetitive exercise at only a modest increase in breathing that can be maintained," was born. Repeated exercise sessions—running, walking, swimming, cycling, dancing, cross-country skiing—create an improved ability to work out harder and longer. Dr. Cooper recorded physiological factors—heart rate, respiratory capacity, blood pressure, and blood lipids—to show that the trained individual not only improved his own factors but was superior to the untrained. The point system for length and severity of workouts, thus derived, defines fitness and correlates directly to coronary risk factors. **It provides everyone with a measure of his or her own mortality along with a goal of fitness. As such, Dr. Cooper created the fitness revolution.**

But this was just the start. The Cooper Clinic, devoted to preventative medicine, wellness, was founded in Dallas. The Cooper Institute for Aerobics Research was organized, long term epidemiological data was gathered, many research grants were received and professional papers published. For over 25 years, coronary risk factors and fitness were measured in repeated tests producing a data base of more than 33,000 individuals. The tests have proven that aerobics has increased the life span among the physically fit and can dramatically decrease the risk factors once the unfit enter an aerobics program.

One indicator that the medical community has accepted the Cooper Clinic's thesis—that physical fitness reduces all-cause mortality—is the publication of study results in the *Journal of the American Medical Association (JAMA)* (Blair, et al., 1989). Deaths in four age groups from

20 to 60 years, for both men and women, were plotted. In each group, death rate decreased strikingly as fitness is increased, most dramatically at ages 50 to 60. This decrease is not great between high fitness categories in the upper quartile, showing that moderate fitness, attainable by briskly walking 30 to 60 minutes each day is sufficient for the training effect. Dr. Cooper has stated for years, *"If you run more than 15 miles per week, you are running for something other than fitness and the emotional balance, good health and good looks that accompany it."* Aerobics books provide point values which compare all forms of exercise. *All can find an exercise that is suitable.*

A later study presented in June 1993 to the International Preventative Cardiology Meeting in Oslo and reported in the *Cooper Clinic Newsletter* shows remarkable results, comparing men who have all three of the traditional high risk factors for coronary disease ... smoking, high blood pressure, and cholesterol. The actual death rates per 10,000 in this group was 124 for the low, 59 for moderate and 30 for the high fitness subgroups. Another striking observation was that high fitness men having traditional coronary risks are actually better off than low fitness men with none of the coronary risk factors, with a death rate of 30 compared to 54 for the latter.

Remember Hans Selye's alarm reaction **"... increased corticoidal activity, increased blood pressure, heart rate and rate of breathing."** These are the precise characteristics improved by Kenneth Cooper's aerobics program. Also remember Hans Selye's stress diversion—**aerobics provides direct stress diversion and trains the cardiovascular system to withstand emergency stress.**

Dr. Cooper has gone on to author a series of books on preventive medicine: *Controlling Cholesterol, Preventing Osteoporosis, It's Better to Believe, Controlling Hypertension,* and his newest, *Advanced Nutritional Therapies*. The thrust of his current efforts is to bring aerobic fitness to all age groups. His research shows that even modest activity can procure substantial benefits. It is not necessary to be an elite athlete to reap benefits.

The Aerobic Conditioned Person:
- With aerobics, the involuntary muscles of the heart, chest and blood vessels are exercised. Isometrics or weight lifting offer little aerobic effect.
- Lung capacity can be doubled.
- Blood volume is increased, hemoglobin, carrying oxygen, is increased as is the blood supply to the heart.
- Greater tissue vascularization is the most remarkable aerobic effect. Arteries increase in size.
- Blood pressure decreases because blood vessels become more pliable.
- The conditioned person can accept the increases in blood pressure and heart rate brought about by physical effort and emotional stress.
- The trained person is relaxed, physically and mentally.
- The digestive system is more relaxed and efficient. Exercise is a natural cathartic.
- Muscle tone, musculature and "build" are all improved.
- Heart rate is dramatically decreased when resting.
- The conditioned heart may sustain 170 to 190 beats per minute for 20 to 30 minutes. An unconditioned person may experience a higher rate, 220 or more beats per minute due to mental or physical stress.
- The conditioned person sleeps well at night and is more "alive" and active through the day.

# 11

# FITNESS FATNESS WELLNESS

In his medical advice columns in *Runners World*, November 1980 and August 1983, Dr. George Sheehan presented the ideal way to lose weight. His basic premise is that one cannot lose fat and maintain fat free weight on diet alone. A classic study by Dr. Ancel Keys of the University of Minnesota showed that a severely restricted 12-week diet resulting in a 25-pound loss, resulted in only an 11-pound fat loss. A second week showed a 6-pound fat loss out of a 9-pound total loss.

Dynamic exercise of the large muscles reduce **body fat**, while retaining and building muscle mass. A diet having modest caloric restrictions, coupled with endurance exercises, will restrain eating habits while building body density.

The thermic effect of exercise is one of Martin Katahn's T-Factors. Metabolism is raised for a considerable time after a workout, and the heart rate may still be elevated the next morning.

The direct correlation between exercise and weight loss is corroborated by a Baylor University long-term study reported in *Runner's World* (Gambaccini, Jan. 1997). In the supervised first year, dieters (without exercise) reduced 15 pounds compared to the exercisers' (without diet) 6 pounds. But in the unsupervised second year, dieters gained back almost all their loss while the exercisers held steady, showing an overall better result, 6 pounds net loss versus 2 pounds. This showed that the exercisers held the line, kept up their new activity, but that dieters slipped back to "normalcy."

Runners have long speculated on the addictive effect of routine workouts, and this would apply to all aerobic activities, including walking. Speculation has it that an increase in endorphins, a morphine-like substance secreted by the pituitary gland, promotes a feeling of whole-body wellness. You simply want to do the daily or tri-weekly workout.

Contrast this with a typical calorie counting diet—you don't feel good at all. Diets that depend on a deprivation which causes a yearning fail in the long run. And this points to the Zone which evens out blood sugar so there is no deprivation.

What about age? Dr. Kenneth H. Cooper has demonstrated that no one is too old to start an exercise program and that walking may be the best exercise. He says, *"You'll be surprised how little activity is necessary ... just avoid inactivity to get substantial health benefits."* An Aerobics Center Longitudinal Study at the Cooper Institute, reported in their April 1994 *Newsletter,* proves that fitness derived from physical activity markedly increases the time period of independent vs. assisted living for the elderly—perhaps, theoretically as much as 10 to 15 years. The study showed that highly fit men and women had about one-third the risk for developing functional limitations than the low fit and that the moderately fit about two-thirds.

Steven Blair, Director of Research at the Cooper Institute for Aerobics Research, wrote the Foreword to the book, *Big Fat Lies* by Glenn Gaesser, stating that extra weight is of "little or no consequence, healthwise—*as long as you are physically fit*" (Gaesser, 1996, p. xvii). And he goes on to say that being thin is no assurance of good health if you are a couch potato. These strong conclusions tell us that exercise is a prime consideration and that slenderness by itself may be merely cosmetic.

This is not a brief for fatness. It is a clarion call for fitness. The *Cooper Newsletter* of Summer 1997 discusses a long-term study at the Cooper Institute for Aerobics Research of 25,000 men followed from 1970. Laura Shapiro's cover story in *Newsweek,* April 21, 1997, "Does It Matter What You Weigh?" showed that fit obese men had a lower risk of death than unfit men of normal weight. But we ask how many fit obese men are there? It does not go with the territory.

The Cooper Clinic of Dallas lists coronary risk factors as fitness, blood pressure, body fat, cholesterol, triglycerides, glucose, and exercise EKG (other than life or lifestyle). We know there is considerable correlation between these risk factors. We should strive for non-obesity, which will lower blood pressure and improve blood factors, *but there is a paramount need to exercise.*

Laura Shapiro's well presented article in *Newsweek* and Glenn Gaesser's book tell us that the obese can still be fit and healthy without yo-yo dieting, as long as they maintain an exercise program. The facts offer a message of hope, and give us good reason to abandon diets that do not work.

The diet suggested by Glenn Gaesser is a 20% fat diet similar to Katahn in Chapter Two. The theme of *Starch Madness* is that this diet, overfeeding high glycemic carbohydrates, *is almost designed to keep the obesity cycle glowing for those of us with Paleolithic genes.*

*The Zone Diet works.*

> *Remember: no matter how modest or lofty your exercise goals, a high-carbohydrate diet may keep you from achieving them. If you're eating too much carbohydrate, you can expect the following, even if you're on a judicious program of aerobic exercise: constant hunger, decreased mental alertness, difficulty in losing body fat (if not out right fat gain), decreased oxygen transfer to the muscle cells, and decreased endurance. All of these are consequences of being out of the Zone* (Sears, 1995, p. 64).
>
> *What will the Zone, this state of optimal health, get you? Even if you're not ill, it will help prevent the likelihood of disease. Many chronic disease conditions such as obesity, heart disease, cancer, diabetes, depression, and alcoholism have a strong genetic linkage. The potential for their expression lies buried in your genetic code. In the Zone, you dramatically decrease the likelihood that those genes will be expressed. The further you are from the Zone, the more likely those genes will be expressed. More immediate, in the Zone you'll have greater access to stored body fat (instead of stored carbohydrate) for energy. You'll also benefit from greater mental concentration, which will not only help you be more productive, but will improve your physical performance as well* (Sears, 1995, p. 37).

The chapter "Exercise in the Zone" from *The Zone* by Barry Sears is required reading. Following the Zone diet preferentially burns body fat for energy (which is why one simply does not experience hunger pangs even with a large daily caloric deficit). When out of the Zone, fat release drops and the body turns to an inferior fuel, carbohydrate. Light aerobic exercise keeps one in the Zone, in runners' parlance—long, slow distance.

> *What's the best exercise to achieve this: (Fat burning) It's called walking. Have you ever wondered why Europeans aren't fat? They don't go to aerobics classes, they just walk a lot.* (Sears, 1995, p. 58).

Paleolithic man was "in shape." Health organizations abound with facilities for people of all ages to obtain strength and endurance training. Shopping malls have opened their doors to all-weather walking. Airports are another great all weather walking area. YMCAs have classes in dance and water aerobics besides all the weight machines and treadmills.

Tables of point values for over forty aerobics exercises and sports are provided in Dr. Cooper's book, *Aerobics Program for Total Well Being*. What could be simpler? Obtain 30 points weekly and you will be in shape, a conditioned person. By no means is running paramount. I attained my top treadmill time five years after ceasing the jarring of running. Dance aerobics for 30 minutes provide 6 points! All of us can find a varied program.

The Schwinn Air-dyne stationary cycle is the inside exercise machine of choice. Both the arms and the legs work contiguously, thus providing more aerobic value per unit of time than almost all other activities or machines. Your energy is dissipated by fan blades, keeping you comfortable, which translates to longer workouts. Its list price is $549.95.

In the business world, as stated by Roy Hurley in 1959 (see page 16), if decisions were made only when there was a 90 percent certainty, little progress would be made. Yet medical science, with the FDA watchdog, seems to operate in that fashion. We should stay abreast of innovations to make considered choices. Case in point—vitamin C. Only now after 30 years has the establishment begun to recognize the need for increasing levels. Another case in point is the evolutionary diet!

The many medical newsletters frequently published by universities and medical institutions provide conservative, carefully documented, proven information. For the cutting edge of wellness reports, I suggest *Health & Healing* monthly report written by Dr. Julian Whitaker (available from Phillips Publishing, 7811 Montrose Road, Potomac, MD 20854, phone 800/777-5005).

For example, I learned about Dr. Batmanghelidj and water from the report. I began to wash my hands thoroughly after another report teaching that personal hygiene improves albumin levels, resisting infection. From an article on the Sonicare toothbrush, which cleanses the gum margins and between the teeth and also halts bad breath, I feel I have a four-year jump on most other users. From the August 1997 report I learned about homocysteine (page 43). Information my wife gleaned about shark cartilage may have averted a serious operation on her ankle. And on and on. And the newest in December 1997: *Yow*, a plaque fighting and scientifically prepared breath freshener that works—it is sold by Target stores.

What "news" is discriminating and what only adds to our confusion? I hope that the wellness and fitness truths from the great minds that have been presented here will permit you to better cope with the often conflicting media pronouncements. From knowledge will come peace of mind. We close the book with an immutable diet primer derived from the Paleolithic understanding.

# 12

# MY DIET PRIMER

What is my "losing weight" diet? What should yours be? This book is mostly a third person report on the great minds of fitness and wellness of the last half century. What then is *my* best advice?

I have found two venues for wellness: the *Zone diet and exercise*. Let me again add the caveat that it is not for me to state that you, personally, should enter into either one. You should consult your best medical advisors, but hopefully this book will provide guidelines for your discussion.

Why bring in exercise? The Zone diet will consume your fat, albeit a bit slower, without exercise. But the two are so serendipitous, so inseparable, that if you can develop the discipline to accomplish the one, you *can* accomplish the other.

> *Remember this: Fitness is a journey, not a destination. That's the secret. It's discipline. The Book of Proverbs says, "Shame and poverty come to those who are not disciplined." I think the secret to success in any field—whether it is fitness, health, or longevity—is discipline. Discipline with your diet, discipline with your weight, discipline with your exercise"* (Cooper, 1995).

The Zone diet levels out your blood sugar, keeping insulin levels even, giving you that Zone feeling. You're not hungry at 10:00 A.M. or craving a cocktail at 5:00 P.M. And a second Zone feeling is provided with exercise. Exercise provides a positive addiction. You will *crave* the next exercise period. This is a feeling hard to describe, but it is so true. With both of these great superman sensations, it is a perfect time to cease other addicting substances or actions. It will work!

Believe, believe Dr. Kenneth Cooper, Adelle Davis, Linus Pauling, Ph.D., Barry Sears, Ph.D., Dr. Fereydoon Batmangheldij, Dr. Hans Selye, Dr. George Sheehan, and all of those others whose research is so convincing. Of course all the diets discussed in this book are designed to accomplish the same purpose. I look for points of similarity and hope to have pointed clearly to points of variation.

This chapter illustrates *my* diet primer. If you wish to "join in," you should determine *your* own diet primer using the Zone tables to determine your nutrient requirements. It is revealing to learn your body make-up and a pleasure to watch the tape measure readings decrease as you enjoy the Zone.

The proportions of protein at 30 percent, carbohydrate at 40 percent, and fat at 30 percent have been discussed in Chapter Five. This works out in gram proportions rather closely to 7/9/3 protein, carbohydrate, and fat (in calories, 28/36/27). *The Zone* book eliminates about 90 percent of laborious counting by providing a convenient "block" method which is applied to your particular meal ration, plus listing the various macronutrient measures in blocks. My meal block is 4.5—4.5 protein, 4.5 carbohydrate and 4.5 fat. My wife's meal block is three. (Each protein block is 7 grams; each carbohydrate block is 9 grams. But each fat block is 1.5 grams, since most protein foods contain entrained fat. Thus the overall 7/9/3 proportion is attained reasonably well.) Once you make up your own primer, using your favorite foods, the system becomes automatic.

Now, the protein daily ration in the Zone diet is essential each day, and I have proven that this is very similar to almost all other "official" diets. The daily fat ration is essential each day, and I have proven that the Zone reducing diet is *very* low fat. The major calorie deficit is from carbohydrate, *but not the carbohydrate necessary for vitamins, fiber, minerals, and the starch necessary for a healthy glucagon to insulin balance.* The unhealthy, empty, starch and sugar calories are gone!

I'll use the Katahn Diet as the exemplar of the Pyramid and/or the *Consumer Reports,* Oct 1992 Ideal Diet, which will be compared to the Zone. If we assume meats as a source of the essential fats and complete protein, we will arrive at about the same absolute quantities by and large, whether we start from the fat side which is Katahn's approach or from the protein side which is Sears' approach. The reason that this Jack Sprat routine works out is that both protein and fat are present in meat, so limiting either one will of course limit the other. There are good and bad choices from either direction so you must, most of the time, pick good choices. These are listed in *The Zone* book, and the Netzer food count book allows you to list and rate your favorite foods.

Table Ten lists protein, fat, and carbohydrate content of a variety of common foods. The meat portions are four ounces, which is close to my meal ration of 4.5 blocks. My wife would cut this down to 3 blocks. These desired meal rations are shown at the top of the table.

Then, at a meal, I add 7 grams of polyunsaturated fat to go along with the entrained fat in the meat, for the overall 30/40/30 relationship. The blocks make this easy. Remember that we learned in Chapter Four that fat in lean beef is 61 percent unsaturated, in fish up to 96 percent unsaturated. Thus my fat intake is easily superior to the

American Heart Association guideline of one-third poly-unsaturated, one third mono-unsaturated, and one third saturated.

## TABLE 10
## Protein and Fat Gram Typical Sources from Netzer Food Counts

|  | Protein | Fat | Carbohydrate (grams) |
|---|---|---|---|
| **My desired meal ration** | **31** | **7** | **41** |
| My wife's desired meal ration | 21 | 4.5 | 28 |
| Beef, lean ground, 4 oz. | 29 | 18 | 0 |
| Beef, round lean only | 33 | 8 | 0 |
| Beef, T-bone lean only | 32 | 12 | 0 |
| Pork, loin lean | 39 | 16 | 0 |
| Veal, leg lean | 41 | 6 | 0 |
| Chicken, white | 35 | 5 | 0 |
| Chicken, dark | 31 | 11 | 0 |
| Turkey, white | 34 | 4 | 0 |
| Turkey, dark | 32 | 8 | 0 |
| Salmon | 24 | 10 | 0 |
| Tuna Steak | 26 | 6 | 0 |
| Tuna, water pack | 26 | 2 | 0 |
| Sword Fish | 29 | 6 | 0 |
| White Fish | 28 | 8 | 0 |
| Trout | 26 | 7 | 0 |
| Yogurt, non fat 8 oz. | 13 | 0 | 16 |
| Yogurt, fruit, 8 oz. | 9 | 3 | 46 |
| Cottage Cheese, nonfat, 8 oz. | 30 | 0 | 10 |
| Cottage Cheese, 2%, 8 oz. | 28 | 5 | 8 |
| Cheddar Cheese, 1 oz. | 6 | 9 | 0 |
| Colby Cheese, 1 oz. | 6 | 9 | 0 |
| Swiss Cheese, 1 oz. | 8 | 8 | 0 |
| Milk, whole, 8 oz. | 8 | 8 | 11 |
| Milk, 2%, 8 oz. | 8 | 4.7 | 11 |
| Milk, 1%, 8 oz. | 8 | 2.7 | 11 |
| Milk, skim, 8 oz. | 9 | 0 | 13 |
| Egg, one whole | 6 | 5 | — |

Now review the make-up of typical fast foods in Table Eleven. I again place meal rations at the top of the table, this time showing total fat ration. Obviously, fast foods should be limited. However, the 4 to 3 relationship between carbohydrate and protein can be maintained quite nicely. You need not be driven out of the Zone.

### TABLE 11
### Macronutrient Gram Make-up for Typical Fast Foods from Netzer Food Counts

|  | Protein | Fat | Carbohydrate | Calories |
|---|---|---|---|---|
| My desired meal ration | 31 | 14 | 41 | 500 max. |
| My wife's desired meal ration | 21 | 9 | 28 | 375 max. |
| McDonalds |  |  |  |  |
|   Big Mac | 25 | 28 | 47 | 530 |
|   McChicken | 17 | 30 | 44 | 510 |
|   Egg McMuffin | 17 | 13 | 27 | 290 |
|   Large Fries | 6 | 22 | 57 | 450 |
| Burger King |  |  |  |  |
|   Big Fish | 26 | 41 | 56 | 700 |
|   Whopper | 27 | 39 | 45 | 640 |
| Wendys |  |  |  |  |
|   Big Bacon Classic | 36 | 33 | 45 | 610 |
|   Grilled Chicken | 24 | 7 | 35 | 290 |
| Pizza Hut |  |  |  |  |
|   Personal Pan Supreme | 33 | 34 | 70 | 720 |
| Hardees |  |  |  |  |
|   Bacon/Egg/Biscuit | 19 | 30 | 45 | 530 |
|   Bacon Cheeseburger | 29 | 34 | 29 | 530 |
|   Grilled Chicken | 23 | 9 | 30 | 290 |
|   Chicken Fillet | 24 | 15 | 46 | 420 |

All of this is intended to give you the "idea" of using the food count book and package labels to build your meals around your favorite foods. Veal, chicken, turkey, and many fish selections comply. Then eat red meat about as often as tuna or sole and you will hit an average. But you also see that when you start out from either fat or protein, you will naturally get the other.

To complete your own diet primer, compile similar tables for carbohydrate foods. You will quickly see how the calories correspond to the "good" and "bad" tables of Montignac and Sears for glycemic index. Starch foods can be eaten, but in limited amounts that curtail your intake of fibers, vitamins, and minerals—thus, not desirable! The mealtime conviviality of dining with family and friends, even the gustatory sensations when eating alone, are partially dependent on the time spent eating and the amount of chewing. Ergo, learn to eat the almost unlimited amount of low glycemic foods, thus keeping you laughing and sparkling at parties instead of fattening up from overeating starches or feeling downtrodden because you can't join in.

The third macronutrient is fat. Fat has been a preoccupation for diet faddists for all of my fifty years of diet study. The true preoccupation should be the 4 to 3 ratio of carbohydrate to protein and the correct "prescription" of protein amount for your body lean weight and activity level. It is insulin triggered by carbohydrate that makes you fat (Sears, 1997, p. 12). Fat is neutral and in fact slows the effects of carbohydrates. Excellent sources of good fats are salad oils and nuts. Remember that most protein foods contain entrained fats, which may be more than 50 percent saturated, so select your added fat in dressings and nuts from those that are unsaturated. And remember the Zone ratios of protein, carbohydrate, and fat, in percent 30/40/

30, in calories 28/36/27, in grams 7/9/3. The Zone block system makes these proportions automatic.

The labels on canned, frozen, and baked foods are now so instructive. For example, I love baked beans, and the protein/fat looks reasonable, but the carbohydrate just throws it out. There is a wide selection of tinned meats and seafood; people buy it for their cats who fare better than their owners. I buy the liquid salad dressings, olive oil, and other unsaturated oils, because you will automatically use a lot less than the viscous type. You don't want the sugar and saturated fat in baked goods and desserts. Of course, we all have our downfalls; Montignac loves dark chocolate. Just try to limit the dessert to a very special treat.

So it does not seem that the absolute amounts of protein and fat in the Sears or the Katahn diets are too much at variance. In my own work-up, I actually would assume about 50 grams fat daily in the Katahn diet and 42 mathematically determined by Sears' procedures. Of course the wild card is carbohydrates.

Another point of similarity is that not eating fat in the Katahn diet rules out desserts, and not eating fats and starches in the Zone rules out desserts. A winner from either direction.

So, with a few adjustments, we would build to either diet. But vital to those 75 percent of us with Paleolithic genes are these Zone precepts (and this goes back to many early teachings of Adelle Davis):

- Protein, fat, and carbohydrate at each meal;
- Equal calories at each meal with no single meal greater than 500 calories;
- Stay away from high glycemic foods, particularly sugar and refined grains.

At this point, I'll delineate my typical day in the Zone diet. To start off, try to find a week when you will be eating at home, or at least for three or four days. Shop the outer aisles for fresh vegetables and fruit.

**BREAKFAST** at 7:30: 8 oz. nonfat plain yogurt, 4 oz. nonfat cottage cheese, plenty of fruit selected from apple, melon, peach, grapes, blueberries, strawberries (need I go on) plus an orange and about seven grams of nuts.

**LUNCH** at 12:30: 3 cups or so mixed vegetable salad, broccoli, red cabbage, cauliflower, cucumber, endive, green pepper, mushroom, onion, tomato (a cornucopia!) with oil & vinegar dressing. (Lawry's makes a nice variety of wine dressings. The dressing is a liquid and excess falls to bottom of bowl.) Protein, usually canned salmon, tuna, chicken. An ounce or so of hard cheese plus 2 ½ Ritz crackers.

**DINNER** at 6:30: Fish such as salmon, swordfish, tuna, or chicken. (My wife has become expert at fixing this sautéed in a Calphalon ripple pan with great seasonings.) Green vegetables, piece of special whole grain bread. Oh yes, two glasses red wine.

So that's simple. My wife only cooks one meal, but you can be as complicated as the very devil. You can get many gourmet recipes from Barry Sears. Usually I don't snack, but the Sears snack bars are great, a cup of 1% milk is okay, even a scoop of Ben & Jerry's when traveling. This totals about 1500-1700 calories.

I included the meal pattern because I don't feel deprived. I'm absolutely in the Zone and feel great. I'm certainly not light-headed as one critic (nasty, nasty) characterized we in the Zone. And, I've been subjected to plenty of 1500-1700 calorie diets that are killers! This aspect of satisfaction is the factor that the critics can't seem to believe. It works, it works, believe, believe!

There is criticism of the Zone described in this book. I have provided a reasoned dismissal of this criticism, I believe, but at least you are made aware of it.

How to make up your particular needs of the macronutrients is beyond the purview of this book. The Barry Sears Zone books provide procedures for each person, male or female, ectomorph or mesomorph, sedentary or active, to determine protein, carbohydrate, and fat needs.

I am 200 lbs. with 160 lbs of lean body mass. The Zone nutrient levels are based on your lean body mass. You can get a relative idea from this book, but buy the Zone book for body mass charts and systems of judging food requirements. One size does not fit all! You will quickly learn the system. You will learn how to eat in restaurants, how to judge protein requirements by the palm of your hand, how to devise a diet using your favorite foods (well, some of them).

It's quite easy to dine out expensively; those $12 to $18 and higher meals can be ordered to follow the Zone very well. You can have a baked potato or a crusty roll, but not both! You can particularly find variety in healthy fish and sea food. When you eat out, try to select gourmet, special foods, treat yourself.

If you presently eat at a fast food place seven days a week, well, STOP! On occasion a chicken or a fish sandwich, a salad, and diet soda will not keep you out of the Zone. You can even find many fast food operations with salad bars. But the salads that are packaged are mostly lettuce which is pretty much devoid of food value, even fiber, and is only a "vehicle" to carry salad dressing. (This applies at home also.)

But you can find really good, rapid service, inexpensive restaurants. In Florida and the southeast, we have Sonny's Real Pit Bar-B-Que. I'll give them an accolade, because they have the absolutely top salad bar plus about six meats that are served sliced or grilled. The salad bar has fresh veggies galore—broccoli, cauliflower, white onion, green onion, tomatoes, green peppers, cucumber. Throw in a few olives and beets for color and I'm in hog heaven. Even a beer for carbohydrate. You know most salad bars: lettuce with half a dozen "pasta, pasta, pasta" salads, not at Sonny's. Of course, if you wish you can have all you can eat ribs, french fries, thick white bread slathered with margarine and fried, baked beans with more meat than beans, cole slaw swimming in dressing. A visit to Sonny's, sticking on the Zone diet, immediately makes you feel like superman. It's your choice!

## DIET TIPS

1. Determine your daily protein requirements using the Zone standard quantities for your lean body mass and your activity level. You will need to buy the Zone book.
2. Select macronutrients in these proportions: 40% carbohydrate, 30% fat, 30% protein.
3. Select non-saturated fats for any added fat over the entrained fat in meat or dairy products that you eat to obtain your protein requirement.
4. Best protein source: salmon, other fish, chicken, turkey.
5. Select carbohydrates from the just about unlimited low glycemic green vegetables.
6. Eat breakfast! Try to eat three equal caloric meals per day (of no more than 500 calories each).
7. Eat the evening meal early, 6:00 p.m. Don't go to bed loaded up, bloated up.

8. Remember the foods that have a double whammy, both sugar and saturated fat, no-nos on all diets, most desserts and sweets.
9. Wean yourself from sugar and sugar substitutes. Why keep yourself in sugar training with ersatz gook.
10. Eat a Zone favorable snack, if hungry between meals (100 calories).
11. Remember that exercise dissipates stress. Without stress, you can diet.
12. Fit your food selections into the precepts of good nutrition by studying the Cooper Clinic "Optimal Nutrition Tip Sheet," reprinted in Appendix Two.

Fine, now what about a lifetime maintenance diet? I'm quite certain that the Zone will function in a healthy fashion in the short term. Certainly my blood profile indicates this. What about the long term?

The research by Dr. Edgar Gordon cited in Chapter 3 tells us that when we, the former obese get our fat down (ideally males 15%, females 25%), we can successfully handle a "regular" diet. I believe that for me a regular diet is the Zone most of the time, with more variety, but I do not want to slip back to fatness. Here are the regular diet words of the great, good and wise patriarch Linus Pauling, writing at age 84. (Pauling also recommends vitamins in greater amounts than those recommended in general in our present antioxidant revolution. I hope that you will get his book, and decide about vitamins for yourself, as this is out of my book's purview. Certainly, I have increased my B-vitamin intake because of our present knowledge about homocysteine.

1. *Keep your intake of ordinary sugar (sucrose, raw sugar, brown sugar, honey) to 50 pounds per year, which is half*

*the present U.S. average. Do not add sugar to tea or coffee. Do not eat high sugar foods. Avoid sweet desserts. Do not drink soft drinks.*
2. *Except for avoiding sugar, eat what you like—but not too much of any one food. Eggs and meat are good foods. Also, you should eat some vegetables and fruits. Do not eat so much food as to become obese.*
3. *Drink plenty of water every day.*
4. *Keep active, take some exercise. Do not at any time exert yourself physically to an extent far beyond what you are accustomed to.*
5. *Drink alcoholic beverages only in moderation.*
6. *Do not smoke cigarettes.*
7. *Avoid stress. Work at a job that you like. Be happy with your family* (Pauling, 1986, p. 9).

# 13

# A CALL TO ARMS

*American Heart Association Scientific Statement*
Ronald M. Krause, et al.,
"Dietary Guidelines for Healthy Americans," Vol. 97, No. 7, 1997
*American Heart Association Scientific Statement*
Alan Chait, et al., "Rationale of the Diet-health Statement
of the AHA," Vol. 88, No. 6, 1993
(obtain AHA information at 800-242-8721)
*Eat Right for (4) Your Type*
Dr. Peter J. D'Adamo with Catherine Whitney
(C.P. Putnam's Sons, 1996)

I have enjoyed reading the American Heart Association (AHA) Scientific Statements listed above. Their Nutrition Committee is made up of the distinguished nutrition experts from our nation's research institutions. A brief history of their recommendations on diet since 1957 is contained in the Vol. 88, No. 6 Report. It is of interest to observe how the various diets discussed in this book mirror the recommendations, and to consider how the commercial food industry has interpreted (or misinterpreted) them.

I am not so presumptuous that I would attempt to compare the Zone diet with the AHA guidelines, but this is exactly what Barry Sears has indirectly done. And he has drawn criticism that I would term superficial since it is so easily refuted. It is largely based on quite casual misunderstanding of the Zone diet. I have discussed this in Chapter Five. The Zone has given me a control over my body that had eluded me for 50 years. I believe I owe it to my own ethic to speak out, to make *a plea directly to the highest diet intellects to prove a reasoned consideration of the Zone precepts.*

- What is the correct amount of daily dietary protein for each lean body mass and activity level?
- Is elevated insulin the primary harbinger of coronary heart disease?
- Can insulin be kept level, keeping blood sugar properly controlled with a carbohydrate/protein proportion? What is the correct proportion?
- Will this insulin level permit the burning of fat without ketosis?
- What are the implications of this insulin level to control or prevent the diseases of civilization?
- What are the absolute amounts of daily dietary fat for each lean body mass and activity level?
- What is the biochemical or hormonal explanation of metabolism? (The nub of the Zone is the critical balance between insulin and glucagon—carbohydrate stimulates insulin, protein stimulates glucagon; Yin and Yang, thus the 4 to 3 ratio between carbohydrate and protein, always companions. Is this an accurate explanation of metabolism?)
- What is the effect of high glycemic foods? (Define complex carbohydrate and refined carbohydrate, and place the basic starch foods into each category.)

- Is the Zone diet healthy as a reducing diet? Does it remain healthy as a life's eating pattern (at which time additional fats are eaten)?

Once this information is gathered, we would have a basis for a critique of the Zone diet *(and all diets)*. Macronutrient meal and daily needs should be stated in absolute terms, not percentages which do not account for life style or activity levels.

*I pray that the American Heart Association will form a committee to document these questions because I believe that Barry Sears' Zone will presage a watershed change in our national diet patterns.*

However, we could easily obtain short-term information safely. In four or six months we could have very solid results. We would want to know actual fat reduction, blood profiles, and stress EKGs. Now you, the reader, if interested, could, with the approval of your doctor, obtain these before-and-after tests and be a study set of one. By all means report to Barry Sears, as have so many others. These results will have a cumulative importance.

I pray that the many wellness institutions throughout the country that combine "sports" medicine and nutrition departments will include a category on their dietary questionnaire that will document the Zone diet. In this way, data will accumulate over a few years without much cost or effort. And for the common good!

I pray that fund managers, foundation managers, and corporate sponsors who read these words will provide monies to respected research institutions to conduct controlled studies. The cost of this simple resolution would be trivial compared to the benefits to all humanity.

Once short-range diet data accumulate, I pray that actual epidemiological studies will be formulated for life's eating pattern proofs. We know that blood lipids tend to normalcy upon weight loss, mine certainly have done so. Will they remain proper on the Zone diet as a life's eating pattern? Sears advises that when normal weight is attained and no further loss is desired, then increase the amount of non-saturated fats. If we over-indulge, then we can remember the Sears dictum that we can readily get back in the Zone at the next meal. But what will happen to those of us who achieve our goal of slenderness and continue the Zone long range? Will additional non-saturated fats be healthy? I believe they will, but would hope to see all of this proven epidemiologically.

I have tried to pose these questions clearly and pray that true scientists will provide considered answers, more than the inexactness of epidemiology. I pray that exacting biochemical explanations can be provided by theorem and verified by experiment.

Dr. Peter J. D'Adamo has written an engaging diet theory in *Eat Right for (4) Your Type*—your individual diet should correlate to your blood type. He points out that blood type O corresponds to the Paleolithic and type A to the age of agriculture, with types B and AB still later mutations. In this book we relate proper diet to our genes and discuss body types (see page 116) which produce the nutrition experts able to cope with high starch diets. Our thesis is that two-thirds of us will profit from the Zone diet. Are we blood type O? I am. Are the type A blood type people able to be slender eating starches?

The work of Dr. D'Adamo certainly tells us that the Pyramid type high-starch diets should not be prescribed for everyone. It is speculation that there may be correlation between obesity, body type, and blood type. But such intriguing speculation. I pray that research institutions will mine their data banks to find out, and that new epidemiological studies will include these protocol.

# 14

# THE WINDUP

Can you afford to wait? We will review those topics central to the new wellness—and to the very old—and ask you the above question. How many did you know about? Which were taught in school? Or in the media?

This book pays rightful homage to the wellness prophets who perceived ahead of their time the essential unity between our diet and daily-life health. Almost to a man they were ignored and in fact often disdained by the scientific community. Most have been poorly reported or not reported at all. Tragic years passed before general acceptance of their breakthrough research.

- *Stress.*   Dr. Selye wrote his treatise on stress control in 1956, but recognized the concept a generation earlier. Now it is general knowledge, but still not widely used as a therapy for family problems, addictions, or overeating.
- *Glycemic index.*   Fifteen years or more after its scientific knowledge, research is being disseminated. This is central to the diets of Montignac and Sears and two-thirds of our population with Paleolithic genes.
- *Saturated fat.*   Analysis of the Paleolithic diet tells us that saturated fat ingestion was low and the p/s ratio

was high. Today's research on circulatory problems tells us to do the same. The Zone diet does this.
- *Protein.* It is essential to eat daily protein amounts in relation to your size and activity level. The Zone gives this information. Other diets may reduce this vital nutrient to an unhealthy degree.
- *Cholesterol.* We have learned that this is not a saturated fat problem, per se, and that the amount of cholesterol we would ingest in the Zone diet and many others is in proportion to the Paleolithic. Of course, the proper approach is to obtain medical advice and before-and-after blood profiles so you can be sure of your own decisions.
- *Water.* The work of Dr. Batmanghelidj is astounding. Is anything so simple and safe with so many possible health results as eight glasses of water daily?
- *Vitamins.* The last great general teaching of Linus Pauling has been his book reviewing the safety and necessity of all the vitamins. Yet he was castigated for twenty-five years for his recommendations on vitamin C. Now, most experts recognize the value of Vitamin C as an antioxidant. Take it, and you will also clear away most colds.

And we have the fascinating lifetime work of Dr. McCully on homocysteine—controlling blood vessel disease with vitamins B6, B12, and folic acid. Again, a wonderful result from simple non-drug products.
- *Aerobics.* Another ho-hum from many a generation ago. Dr. Cooper has been honored worldwide after his absolute proof of its effectiveness in bettering lifestyle and life-span. Now Dr. Cooper has proven that simple walking, which almost all can do at any age, helps greatly.
- *Paleolithic diet.* Barry Sears provides the nutrient proportions of early man, lucidly explaining the intricate metabolism of food and unifying food as the best medicine for curing and preventing disease. The Zone makes the Law of Conservation of Energy operable. At long last,

*food in* plus *body fat—equals—energy out* and the deficit of *weight loss*. Sears also is criticized, but his theorems ring so true!

*Can you afford to wait?*

We've written about Roy Hurley's diet in Chapter Two and listed the "no-nos" to illustrate that, between 1959 and today, we have come full circle. His "diet" had many of the attributes of the Zone ... protein, fat, and carbohydrate at each meal; hearty breakfast; limited saturated fats. He tells us how great he felt, and attributed that Zone feeling to the big breakfast.

There is a picture of Roy Hurley, this 62-year-old executive, a little less fit than at 22, but still down to 186 lbs. with cholesterol of 160 (down from 300), looking like a man in the Zone.

In Chapter Five we have the story Adelle Davis wrote about another man in the Zone, who felt and looked great, and whose diet included protein, fat, and sugarless carbohydrate at every meal.

Barry Sears alludes, in both his Zone books, to an eating pattern taught by your grandmother. Adelle Davis, who indicted starch as our major source of hidden "sugar" forty years before the scientific evidence of glycemic index, is everyone's grandmother. My own maternal grandparents lived to be 88, but only 2 of their 11 children equal this. Forty years before Adelle Davis, we were derailed by manufactured foods designed for shelf life with sugar, salt, and hydrogenated fats. Forty years after Adelle Davis we've been derailed by the "cholesterol in food, cholesterol in the bloodstream" syndrome and by "pasta, pasta, pasta, eating (what was mistermed) complex carbohydrates," starches that Grandmother Adelle Davis knew to add to the sugar deluge. Barry Sears gives us a grim statistic: *Americans on average between 1960-1980 have added 32% more body fat.*

In a January 1994 article, "Pyramid Power," Raymond Sokolov, long-time food writer for *Natural History* magazine, advised the rationale of the USDA to abandon the four basic food groups system of nutrition in favor of the food pyramid. Of course, the thrust of this book is that *both* these diets are skewed against the larger portion of the population. After reading *The Zone,* I no longer feel in the minority, but the Food Pyramid is still a majority position, almost the law of the land, trumpeted happily by most processed food producers. Pasta, pasta, pasta, ad infinitum.

I know that the majority opinion has kept me obese all my life, or struggling to live within the "food-in vs. energy-out" strait-jacket. The ultimate logic for Raymond Sokolov came from a long-term Chinese-American (Cornell University) study investigating the diet of 6500 rural Chinese men, who had much fewer heart problems than the American controls. Further analysis, cited by Barry Sears, tells us, however, that urban Chinese men, who have less exercise but eat the same rice and minimal protein as their rural brethren, have about the same incidence of heart problems as Americans. Ditto Chinese women. Isn't epidemiology wonderful?

There's another factor. Most diet-fitness experts, by the very nature that function follows form, are ectomorphs (lean types). They are in that fortunate 25% (for their insulin production as we now know from the Stanford study cited by Sears) of the population that is not impelled to overeat from starch and sugar ingestion, or whose eicosanoids production is not made awry by high glycemic foods. They feel good anyway. They simply cannot relate to us mesomorphs (broad, stocky muscular types) or endomorphs (round) who have Paleolithic genes and who are by far in the majority.

Think about it. The Jane Fondas of this world present dance aerobics. Dr. Kenneth Cooper, a personal hero and a svelte 160 lbs. innately believes "weight loss is calories-in vs. calories-out" (the Zone now makes this work). The late Dr. George Sheehan, 160 lbs., another personal hero (well, I was a runner for 12 years until my knees could no longer cope with my mesomorphic physique) extols the runner whose exercise keeps his ectomorphic body slender as proof that exercise should do the job for us all. Tell this to Reggie White and other NFL linemen. Martin Katahn (at 5'10", weight 160 lbs.) ignores glycemic index completely in his 1989 book and tells us that all can profit from *Eat, eat, carbohydrates* except those with a *metabolic abnormality*. Roy Walford looks to be about 160 lbs. and lives very well on 60% carbohydrate in his book, *The 120-Year Diet*. These ectomorphs have become the fitness experts because they *look* but more importantly *feel* the part. Calorie counting and high starch diets work for them.

And the word is **eicosanoids**.

**The most persuasive epidemiological evidence is provided by the diet of early man and his precursors, over two billion years, which Barry Sears points out, go back to eicosanoid production in primordial sponges.**

The Zone diet is the easiest eating program that this five-decade diet expert has followed. It accesses fat for energy while providing the necessary macro- and micronutrients to preserve lean body mass (LBM). And, you do not experience hunger or cravings.

For the eons during which the Age of Agriculture is an incidental blip, man ate a low glycemic, protein rich diet. The rarity of sugar and salt appears to be a correlation to which today's researchers should pay attention. Meats having the same level of cholesterol as today's farm-raised red meats were low in saturated fat. In fact, even in the

> *Modern analysis of Neo-Paleolithic diets makes it apparent why our ancestors were so physically developed. First of all, their carbohydrate sources—fruits and fiber-rich vegetables—were exceptionally rich in micronutrients (vitamins and minerals). In fact, it's been estimated recently that the typical diet of Neo-Paleolithic man supplied two to five times the RDA of vitamins and minerals.*
>
> *Far more important, though—and this was reported in a 1985 article in the New England Journal of Medicine—is the fact that almost to the percentage point Neo-Paleolithic diets have the same protein-to-carbohydrate ratio as a Zone-favorable diet. So the Neo-Paleolithic diet kept insulin, glucagon, and eicosanoid responses on an even keel* (Sears, 1995, p. 101).

Age of Agriculture, cholesterol did not appear as a problem until the drastic increase in the use of sugar.

The whole rather paradoxical subject of cholesterol has been reviewed. For state-of-the-art information on this topic the reader is urged to read Kilmer McCully, Linus Pauling, Dallas Clouatre, and Barry Sears. The new research on homocysteine blood levels may alter this whole subject *(see Chapter Four)*. Cholesterol may be an effect, not a cause.

We must stop fitting all pegs in the same hole. We must recognize that there are three basic body types: lean, round, and broad. Without doubt, Katahn's *eat, eat, carbohydrate diet* works for a good portion of people, but we must recognize that for about 65% of us, it creates low blood sugar and the urge to overeat, an urge that transcends discipline.

The Montignac diet "works" because it puts you in the Zone a greater part of the time. I was pleased to discover that the Montignac diet is an advantageous diet when eating out ... easy to follow and satisfyingly rich. Correspondingly, his Maintenance diet works well at cocktail parties. Once you gain the palate for red wines, you can actually look forward to social activities that almost always involve eating and drinking. You are losing weight while enjoying the soiree, which on other diets can be grim. Michel Montignac provides a great deal of practical information on how to cope with the real world of parties and restaurants. His diet becomes the Zone Maintenance Diet.

It is now apparent why the Pyramid diet doesn't work for the two-thirds of us with Paleolithic genes. As a reducing diet, it is inadequate in protein and too high in carbohydrate. We have shown that the absolute amounts of protein in the Pyramid maintenance diet are essentially equal to the absolute amounts in the Zone. However, when the Pyramid diet is used as a reducing diet, the high proportions of carbohydrate are maintained. Then, if calories are cut 30%, protein (which is just adequate in the Pyramid maintenance diet) is also cut 30%, falling too low for good health. As a maintenance diet, as an ideal diet for everyone, it should not be pushed on us Paleolithic types. It impels one to overeat unless the high glycemic food, the foods that are calorically dense and poor in fiber and range of nutrients, are omitted.

The excess insulin produced by the Pyramid diet causes fat cells to develop a resistance to the release of fat while it lowers blood sugar. It *increases* fat stores—the Zone *uses* fat stores. Slowly, after a few servings of bread, rice, pasta, breakfast cereal, and dessert at a time, we Paleolithic people gain back the weight we laboriously lost on calorie counting diets. Barry Sears has given us a *method*, a "leitmotiv," of normality and good health.

It is important to exercise! The Zone diet gives you half the program, but exercise gives you the other. This, too, is

Paleolithic, having a fit body. An emaciated dieter looks bad and almost always fills in again ... with fat. The smart way is to lose weight slowly ... or even gain if the gain is in muscle mass. Do not enter into a calorie counting pyramid type diet if you are exercising heavily. You may be cutting protein and fat dangerously low. The Montignac diet and certainly the quantified Zone diet gives you these vital nutrients.

Dr. Cooper provides us a quantitative indication of our own mortality. His aerobic system correlates directly with health fitness. Dr. Selye's brilliant analysis of stress proves the value of physical activity to mental health. Rudyard Kipling wrote of the Law of the Jungle, *"For the strength of the Pack is the Wolf and the strength of the Wolf is the Pack."* Exercise for fit bodies and fit minds, discipline in diet and stress control—in the words of Kipling, *"The law runneth forward and back."* Accomplish one and you will accomplish the others.

The "diseases of civilization" are diseases that are treated but often not cured. Dr. Batmanghelidj has shown us how they can be mimicked by the lack of water. But consider how they are caused by the modern age of agriculture diet. Amazingly, 8 glasses of water a day may be an answer. In doing this you will find your urge for coffee or cola or beer much less. It works! And in working, it may remove health problems.

I believe that the books reviewed here should be in everyone's lexicon. They are a distillation of the great minds of our era and provide the timeless themes for temporal living. And they mesh together, each feeds on and adds to the others.

You could, for about $210, purchase all of the books listed, and you should. Together with the moral teachings of the Bible, you would have the temporal teachings of wellness, fitness, and discipline.

All right, let us review my reducing diet that works, and issue a challenge to the critics to truly prove a flaw. It is the Stone Age diet revisited—the Zone. Just like Paleolithic man, I eat little saturated fat or refined carbohydrate, and macronutrient proportions are *from the distant past*. It is protein adequate; it provides a procedure that allows anyone to determine their protein needs, without guess work. It provides all the macronutrients for robust health in a ratio that keeps insulin at a level that accesses body fat. (This is the alchemy of it all.) It has by far the healthiest quantities of natural vitamins, minerals, and fibers. And it absolutely, positively, without a doubt, gives you that Zone feeling. You don't know you're on a diet until your clothes need taking in. You sneer at those who need that coffee/coke, doughnut break, smoke, or crave that cocktail; it makes you feel like a superior being.

That said, what about the Zone as a life's eating pattern? First, I hope that this book will engender true epidemiological studies in a big way. Meanwhile, the Zone precepts endure. Two powerful teachings counsel us on the proper attitude toward food. Sears advises us that "no natural substance is entirely good or entirely bad," and Linus Pauling tells us "except for avoiding sugar, eat what you like—but not too much of it!" Moderation. Avoid fad diets. When our body fat is down to normal, we can eat what we like, but not too much.

*The greatest fad diet is the sugar, refined starches, and saturated fat of the age of agriculture.* Stand back to contemplate evolution. Barry Sears has given us the diet proportions of today's food to the Paleolithic; Linus Pauling has given us the vitamins to equal the Paleolithic diets; Kenneth Cooper has given us the robust body of the Paleolithic. It is your decision.

The goal of us all at whatever age is to achieve and enjoy a lifestyle that will enhance our living for tomorrow.

These themes of *Starch Madness* will let us all ask, as did baseball's ageless "Satchel" Page, *"How old would you be if you didn't know how old you were?"*

And finally, an admonition. During an examination at the Mayo Clinic, I indicated my admiration for Adelle Davis, only to learn that my physician, when an intern at a University of Chicago hospital, had been present at her death from cancer, one day after she entered the hospital. She had treated herself with diet. Perhaps the prostate cancer of Dr. George Sheehan could have been discovered with routine physical examinations. None of the wellness tenets discussed in this book can substitute for thorough medical treatment, but hopefully will result in healthy reports.

Postscript: As I write this, my weight is 200 pounds, exactly as it was, redistributed, 56 years ago. Of greater import is my knowledge that I'm in control. I'm in the Zone. You, too, can be!

Richard L. Heinrich
4 Live Oak
Amelia Island, FL 32034

# APPENDIX 1

# FAT-CHOLESTEROL LIST

*The Balancing Act Nutrition and Weight Guide*
by Georgia Kostas, MPH, RD, LD
Copyright. 1993, reprinted by permission.

Use this guide to eat less total fat, saturated fat, and cholesterol.

Daily Goals: 20-30 grams fat (women) or 30-60 grams fat (men)—for weight loss
50 grams fat (women) or 70 grams fat (men)—for weight maintenance
100-300 mg cholesterol
10-15 grams saturated fat
or the advice of your physician or registered dietitian

| FOOD | Serving Size | Cholesterol (milligrams) | Saturated Fat (grams) | Total Fat (grams) |
|---|---|---|---|---|
| Egg | 1 | 213 | 1.5 | 6 |
| Liver, beef | 3 ounce | 370 | 3.5 | 9 |
| Beef, pork, lamb (lean) | 3 ounce | 75 | 3.5 | 8 |
| Veal, lean | 3 ounce | 90 | 2.5 | 5 |

| FOOD | Serving Size | Cholesterol (milligrams) | Saturated Fat (grams) | Total Fat (grams) |
|---|---|---|---|---|
| Chicken, turkey (light meat without skin) | 3 ounce | 60 | 1.3 | 3 |
| Fish | 3 ounce | 45 | .1 | 2.5 |
| Oysters, clams, crab | 3 ounce | 120 | .1 | 2.1 |
| Shrimp (15 med.), lobster | 3 ounce | 95 | .2 | 1.0 |
| Frankfurter, all beef | 1 | 32 | 6.5 | 17 |
| Cold cuts | 3 ounce | 75 | 6.5 | 21 |
| Cheese, American or cheddar | 1 ounce | 25 | 6.0 | 10 |
| Cheese, mozzarella (part skim) | 1 ounce | 15 | 3.0 | 5 |
| Cheese, cottage (1% fat) | 1 cup | 5 | 1.5 | 2.5 |
| Cheese, ricotta (part skim) | 1 cup | 40 | 6.0 | 10 |
| Cream cheese (2 Tbs.) | 1 ounce | 30 | 5.0 | 10 |
| Milk, whole | 1 cup | 35 | 5.0 | 8 |
| Milk, skim | 1 cup | 5 | 0 | 2.5 |
| Yogurt, low-fat | 8 ounce | 15 | 2.5 | 6 |
| Yogurt, nonfat | 8 ounce | 5 | 0.0 | 0 |
| Ice cream | 1 cup | 55 | 8.0 | 18 |
| Ice milk | 1 cup | 15 | 3.0 | 6 |
| Butter | 1 tablespoon | 35 | 7.0 | 14 |
| Margarine, tub | 1 tablespoon | 0 | 2.0 | 11 |
| Oil, vegetable | 1 tablespoon | 0 | 0.0 | 14 |

**Note:** Not all foods are high in both cholesterol and saturated fat. Cut down on foods containing large amounts of **either.**

# APPENDIX 2

# OPTIMAL NUTRITION

The Cooper Clinic Nutrition Program
by Georgia Kostas, MPH, RD, LD, etal.
The Cooper Clinic, Dallas, Texas
Copyright, Rev. 1997, reprinted by permission.

## GUIDELINES FOR OPTIMAL NUTRITION

1. Combine healthy eating with exercise to attain and maintain a healthy body weight.
2. Balance your intake of protein, complex carbohydrates, and fat for well-balanced meals. Combine P-C-F at each meal.

| NUTRIENT | % OF CALORIES | EAT DAILY |
|---|---|---|
| Protein | 10–20% | 4–8 oz. fish, poultry, lean meat, dried peas/beans and<br>2–3 cups skim or low-fat milk/yogurt (or 2 oz. low-fat cheese) |
| Complex Carbohydrate | 50–70% | 5–9 fruit & vegetables, at least 2 raw, and<br>4–11 starches, at least 2 wholegrain |
| Fat | 20–30% | 3–8 tsp. added fats (margarine, oil, dressing)<br>Eat only baked, broiled food—not fried. |
| Water | | 4 glasses (1 qt.) minimum and<br>1 qt. other fluids |

3. Choose a wide food variety at each meal to maximize nutrient variety.
4. Choose fresh, wholesome, unprocessed foods.
5. Establish consistent eating patterns, i.e., 3 meals a day. This promotes sound nutrition, reduces stress, and prevents over-eating. Do not skip meals ... particularly breakfast.
6. Choose more complex carbohydrates (at least 3 per meal) for vitamins, minerals, energy, fiber, and water. Eat fresh fruits and vegetables, wholegrained and enriched cereals (bread, cereals, rice, pasta, grits, oatmeal, cracked wheat, bran), potatoes, corn, peas, beans, lentils, popcorn, pretzels.
7. Choose more dietary fiber (at least 8 fiber foods daily) for good digestion, prevention of digestive diseases, and lowering blood sugar and cholesterol. Fiber is in: bran, whole grains, raw fruits and vegetables (including peels and seeds), nuts, popcorn, beans, brown rice, oatmeal, potatoes, corn.
8. Choose fewer foods high in fat. These include: fried foods, butter, margarine, mayonnaise, oils, sauces, salad dressings, nuts, avocado, granola, party crackers and dips, chips and dips, convenience foods, commercial pastries, high-fat meat (bacon, sausage, cold cuts, hot dogs, marbled beef, lamb, pork), high-fat dairy products (whole milk, sour or sweet cream, cheese, ice cream). Eat more fish, poultry, and veal (10+ meals/week) in place of beef, lamb, pork, and low-fat cheeses (4 meals/week).
9. Choose polyunsaturated and monounsaturated fats in place of saturated fats whenever possible. *Saturated fats are usually animal fats,* found in dairy and meat products, but *sometimes are vegetable fats,* as in chocolate (cocoa butter), coconut, and palm oils. *Polyunsaturated fats* are primarily found in *vegetable* sources: unhydrogenated peanut butter, safflower, corn, sunflower, soybean, sesame, and cottonseed oils, margarines, and fish.

*Monounsaturated fats* are found in olives, peanuts, avocados, some nuts, and olive, canola, and peanut oils.

10. Eat less protein ... just 4-8 oz./day of fish, poultry, and lean meat.
11. Eat less cholesterol ... less than 300 mg/day. Limit these: egg yolks, organ meats, crawfish, meat and meat products, and dairy products (whole milk, sour or sweet cream, cheese, ice cream, butter).
12. Eat less sugar ... Limit sweets to 1-3 weekly. Sugar is in: table sugar, honey, jam, jelly, soft drinks, desserts, candy, cookies, cakes, pastries, processed foods and beverages, sweetened juices and fruit, sugar-coated cereals, peanut butter containing sugar.
13. Limit sodium ... to less than 4000 mg/day. Sources are: salt, pickles, olives, luncheon meats, hot dogs, ham, bacon, sausage, cheeses, processed foods, fast foods, snack foods (chips, crackers, pretzels), canned soups and vegetables, sauces (chili, barbecue, soy, steak), pizza, commercial bakery products.
14. Limit caffeine (a stimulant) to 0-2 cups caffeine-beverages daily. Caffeine is in: coffee, tea, cola drinks, chocolate.
15. Limit alcohol as your doctor directs. At most, limit to 1-2 drinks/day. A "drink" = 1½ oz. liquor, 4 oz. wine, 12 oz. light beer, 8 oz. regular beer = 100 calories.
16. Drink at least 8 glasses of fluids daily, *4 of which are water.*
17. Enjoy your meals! Eat slowly in a relaxed environment. This aids digestion and weight control. *Find ways to deal with stress effectively, without food or alcohol.*
18. Adjust your food intake according to your special needs (i.e., hypertension, high cholesterol levels, diabetes, etc.).

## NUTRIENT GUIDE

CALORIES
>WHY: Energy from food. Adequate calories are necessary to sustain life processes and provide energy; excesses are stored as fat.
>SOURCE: All foods, beverages, alcohol.

PROTEIN
>WHY: Incorporated in all body tissues and organs, bones, muscle, hormones, and enzymes. Regulates acid-base balance. Helps disease resistance.
>SOURCE: Dried beans and peas, fish, poultry, veal (10 meals/week), lean meat (4 meals/week), low-fat dairy products, eggs (3 per week).

COMPLEX CARBOHYDRATE
>WHY: Chief, most efficient energy source. Supplies essential fiber. Spares protein as an energy source. Rich in vitamins and minerals.
>SOURCE: Fresh fruits/vegetables, wholegrain bread/cereals—with bran, oats, wheat, corn, rye, barley, oatmeal, legumes (pinto beans, lentils), starches (potatoes, rice, pastas), popcorn, pretzels (unsalted).

FAT
>WHY: Long-term energy stores. Contain essential fatty acids for skin and health. Carry fat-soluble vitamins.
>SOURCE: Polyunsaturated (vegetable fats)—safflower, corn, sunflower oil, tub margarine, mayonnaise, salad dressing (Italian, French); or monounsaturated fats—olive, canola, or peanut oil.

CHOLESTEROL
>WHY: Precursor of vitamin D and many vital body compounds and component of hormones and cell walls. Excesses deposit in artery walls and may lead to atherosclerosis.

SOURCE: Eggs, organ meats, meat, poultry, fish, shellfish, pork, butter, whole milk dairy products (cheese, ice cream, sweet/sour cream, dips, creamy dressings, etc.).

SUGAR (Simple Carbohydrate)
WHY: High-calorie source but devoid of vitamins and minerals.
SOURCE: Sugar, brown sugar, honey, jam, jellies, soft drinks, candy, cookies, pastries, cake, sugar-coated cereals, other sweets.

ALCOHOL
WHY: A drug and high-calorie source, devoid of vitamins/minerals.
SOURCE: Beer, wine, liquor.

CAFFEINE
WHY: Stimulant—may cause insomnia, irregular heart beat, nervousness, irritant—may increase stomach acidity. Diuretic, muscle relaxant. May aggravate fibrocystic breast disease.
SOURCE: Coffee, tea, cola drinks, chocolate. Over 200 mg/day (2 cups coffee) may have adverse effects.

WATER
WHY: Vital to normal body processes. Temperature control, waste excretion, digestion and absorption of nutrients.
SOURCE: At least 4 (8 oz.) glasses daily and at least 4 of other beverages.

FIBER
WHY: Aids/promotes good digestion, reduces constipation, prevents/treats diverticulosis, decreases risk of colon cancer.
SOURCE: Wheat, bran, wholegrain bread and cereals, fresh fruit/vegetables, beans, nuts, seeds, popcorn, peels, potatoes—8/day minimum.

**CALCIUM**
  WHY: Strong bones, teeth, nails. Muscle tone, prevents cramping. Blood clotting, nerve function. Heart beat, prevents osteoporosis.
  SOURCE: Low-fat dairy products (milk, yogurt, cheese, etc.), dark green leafy vegetables (broccoli, spinach, etc.). Eat at least 2-3 low-fat dairy products daily.

**PHOSPHORUS**
  WHY: Growth and maintenance of strong bones and teeth. Energy production, regulates blood chemistry and internal processes.
  SOURCE: Lean meat, fish, poultry, low-fat dairy products.

**MAGNESIUM**
  WHY: Energy production, normal heart rhythm. Muscle/nerve function, prevents muscle cramps.
  SOURCE: Wholegrain cereals, nuts, legumes, seafood, dark green leafy vegetables.

**SODIUM**
  WHY: Normal water balance inside and outside cells. Blood pressure regulation. Electrolyte and chemical balance.
  SOURCE: In processed foods (ham, bacon, deli meats, cheeses, crackers, pickles, sauces, soups, fast foods, pizza).

**POTASSIUM**
  WHY: Balance and volume of body fluids. Prevent muscle cramping, weakness. Normal heart rhythm. Electrolyte balance in blood.
  SOURCE: Citrus fruits, bananas, green leafy vegetables, potatoes, tomatoes, wholegrains and bran, yogurt.

**ZINC**
  WHY: Appetite, taste acuity, growth, healthy skin, wound healing. Structural part of cells in body.

SOURCE: Lean meat, liver, low-fat milk, fish, poultry, shellfish, wholegrain cereals.

**IRON**
WHY: Formation of red blood cells. Oxygen transport to cells. Prevents nutritional anemia.
SOURCE: Liver, lean meats, legumes, eggs, dark green leafy vegetables, wholegrain cereals, dried fruit.

**VITAMIN A**
WHY: Normal vision, healthy eyes. Prevents night "blindness." Healthy skin, mucous membranes. Resistance to infection. Tissue growth and repair.
SOURCE: Liver, dark green or yellow-orange fruit/vegetables (spinach, carrots, broccoli, cantaloupe, apricots, plums, tomatoes).

**VITAMIN D**
WHY: Promotes calcium and phosphorus absorption; normal growth; healthy bones, teeth, nails.
SOURCE: Vitamin D is formed by action of sunlight on skin. Low-fat dairy products fortified with vitamin D.

**VITAMIN E**
WHY: Prevents spoilage of fats. Preserves foods. Protects cell membranes.
SOURCE: Vegetable oils, margarine. (You need 3 teaspoons daily.)

**THIAMIN ($B_1$)**
WHY: Energy production; appetite; digestion; functioning of nerves, heart, muscle; growth; fertility.
SOURCE: Pork, liver, meat, enriched and fortified wholegrain, legumes, nuts.

**RIBOFLAVIN ($B_2$)**
WHY: Energy production; good vision; healthy skin and mouth tissue.
SOURCE: Low-fat dairy products, lean meat, liver eggs, enriched and fortified wholegrains, green leafy vegetables.

NIACIN ($B_3$)
    WHY: Energy production; healthy skin, tongue; digestive and nervous system; appetite, digestion.
    SOURCE: Fish, lean meats, pork, poultry; liver, nuts, legumes, enriched and fortified wholegrains.

PYRIDOXINE ($B_6$)
    WHY: Energy production; red blood cell formation; growth.
    SOURCE: Pork, liver, lean meats, fish, legumes, enriched and fortified wholegrain, green leafy vegetables.

PANTOTHENIC ACID
    WHY: Energy production; growth and maintenance of body tissues.
    SOURCE: Eggs, lean meats, liver, low-fat milk, wholegrain, legumes, potatoes.

FOLIC ACID
    WHY: Red blood cell formation; energy production
    SOURCE: Green leafy vegetables, liver, lean meat, fish, legumes, nuts, wholegrains.

VITAMIN $B_{12}$
    WHY: Healthy nerve tissue; normal red blood cell formation; utilization of folic acid; energy production
    SOURCE: Liver, lean meat, poultry, fish, eggs, low-fat dairy products.

VITAMIN C
    WHY: Promotes growth, wound healing; resists infection, bone, teeth formation/repair; increases iron absorption.
    SOURCE: Citrus fruits, cantaloupe, strawberries, potatoes, tomatoes, green vegetables (greens, broccoli, cabbage, kale, collards).

Note: The following are nutrient-dense foods, but high in cholesterol (liver, eggs) and fat (nuts, seeds).

## GUIDELINES FOR WEIGHT CONTROL

1. Refuse second helpings.
2. Eat smaller portions of all foods.
3. Double your intake of fresh vegetables and fruit, especially raw.
4. Choose "crunchy" foods ... apples, salads, popcorn, toast, vegetables.
5. Eat less protein: just 4-8 oz./day of meat, fish, poultry, veal.
6. Reduce alcohol consumption.
7. Reduce sweets (candy, soft drinks, desserts, sweet rolls, sugar, etc.).
8. Reduce fats (margarine, mayonnaise, salad dressings, sauces, fatty meats, fast foods, fried foods).
9. Plan healthy snacks.
10. Drink at least 8 glasses of fluids daily.
11. Exercise more.
12. Remember: 3500 calories = 1 pound fat ... Therefore, to lose weight, adjust your calorie intake and expenditure as follows:

| CALORIES<br>Food  Exercise | CALORIES<br>Saved daily | CALORIES<br>Saved weekly | LOSE<br>Weekly |
|---|---|---|---|
| ↓250 + ↑250 = | 500 | 3500 = | 1 pound |
| ↓750 + ↑250 = | 1000 | 7000 = | 2 pounds |

## A BALANCED MENU

| 20% PROTEIN | 55% CARBOHYDRATE (1700 CALORIES) | 25% FAT |
|---|---|---|

BREAKFAST
    ½ cup orange juice     1 small banana
    1 cup skim milk     2 glasses water
    1 cup bran flakes

LUNCH
    Turkey sandwich:     carrot sticks
        2 oz. turkey     1 small orange
        2 slices wholewheat bread     12 pretzels (small twist)
        lettuce, tomato     1 cup skim milk
        2 tsp. mayonnaise

DINNER
    3 oz. broiled fish     Tossed dinner salad
        w/1 tsp. olive oil         w/1 Tbsp. dressing
    1 large baked potato         (French, Italian,
        w/2 tsp. margarine or         oil/vinegar)
        w/3 Tbsp.     ½ cup mixed fresh fruit
            grated low-fat cheese     2 glasses water
    ½ cup steamed broccoli
    ½ cup steamed cauliflower

# APPENDIX 3
# SUGGESTED READING LIST

Total List Prices: $213.53

Batmanghelidj, Dr. Fereydoon. (1992). *Your Body's Many Cries for Water*. Global Health Solutions 800/759-3999. $14.95. You will forevermore drink enough water when you understand its value.

Clouatre, D. & Rosenbaum, M. (1994). *The Diet and Health Benefits of HCA*. New Canaan, CT: Keats Publishing. $3.95. A "natural food" diet aid.

Clouatre, Dallas. (1993). *Getting Lean with Anti-fat Nutrients*. San Francisco: Pax Publishing. $7.95. A well-written statement of diet facts and aids.

Cooper, Dr. Kenneth H. (1982). *The Aerobics Program for Total Well-Being*. Bantam Books. $16.95. The road to fitness by the inventor of aerobics, with point charts for repetitive exercises that will define fitness.

Cooper, Dr. Kenneth H. (1996). *Advanced Nutritional Therapies*. Thomas Nelson, Inc. $24.99. A highly esteemed medical doctor's statement on micronutrients and diet "aids."

Davis, Adelle. (1954). *Let's Eat Right to Keep Fit*. Penguin Books. $5.99. This is your grandmother's nutrition book.

Katahn, Martin. (1989). *T-Factor Diet*. Bantam Books. $6.99. The diet that works for ectomorphs.

Kostas, Georgia G. *The Balancing Act, Nutrition and Weight Guide.* ISBN: 0-9635969-1-8. 972/239-7223. $29.95. A large format handbook of diet and nutrition, well-conceived and presented.

McCully, Dr. Kilmer S. (1997). *Homocysteine Revolution.* Keats Publishing. $14.95. A unified theory of blood vessel disease that may defeat this scourge.

Montignac, Michel. (1991). *Dine Out and Lose Weight.* Montignac USA, Inc., 800/932-3229. $19.95. The first great diet plan to defeat high glycemic carbohydrates.

Netzer, Corinne T. (1997). *Complete Book of Food Counts.* Dell Books. $9.50. 770 pages of food facts.

Pauling, Linus. (1986). *How to Live Longer and Feel Better.* Avon Books. $6.50. The great teachings of our nation's patriarch.

Sears, Barry with Bill Lawren. (1995). *The Zone, A Dietary Road Map.* Regan Books. $25.00. The diet that works for us who need it most.

Selye, Dr. Hans. (1976). *The Stress of Life.* McGraw-Hill Book Co. $12.95. Learn to recognize stress, understand it, and defeat it.

Sheehan, Dr. George. (1989). *Personal Best.* Rodale Press. $14.95. The philosopher of fitness writes about the relationships and understanding of life.

# GLOSSARY

(Words not defined in a standard dictionary)

**Aerobics.** Repetitive exercise at only a modest increase in breathing that can be maintained.

**Amino Acid.** An organic compound that serves as a unit of structure for proteins and is necessary for metabolism.

**Ascorbate.** A salt of ascorbic acid, such as calcium ascorbate or sodium ascorbate. The same vitamin C but with a neutral taste. Many in the "business" do not even know of this version of "C," so much easier to ingest.

**Cholesterol.** Fat-like substance found in blood. Levels broken down to low density lipoprotein (LDL) and high density lipoprotein (HDL).

**Corticoids.** Hormones of the adrenal gland (adrenaline).

**Ectomorph.** Slender, small-boned, physical type. Probably can use calorie diets successfully.

**Eicosanoid.** A "super" hormone. Read Barry Sears on this. The balance of "good" and "bad" eicosanoids is maintained by the 4 to 3 ratio of carbohydrate to protein. Glucagon promotes the "good"; insulin promotes the "bad." Protein maintains glucagon; carbohydrate increases insulin.

**Endomorph.** Round or pear-shaped physical type.

**Epidemiology.** Statistical study of the variable factors or conditions in the cause of disease or health states.

**FDA.** Food and Drug Administration

**Glucagon.** Hormone of the pancreas that restores blood sugar levels and balances the action of insulin.

**Glucose.** Blood sugar. Insulin drives down blood sugar, glucagon restores it. The critical balance between the two (carbohydrate stimulates insulin, protein stimulates glucagon) depends on the 4 to 3 ratio of the Zone and the *size* of the meal (Sears, 1995, p. 28).

**Glycemic index.** The blood glucose response (blood sugar) to a carbohydrate food, expressed as a percentage of the response to the same amount of carbohydrate from a standard food (either glucose or white bread). Entry rate of a carbohydrate into the blood stream.

**Glycogen.** Carbohydrate stored in the liver, which is changed into blood glucose (blood sugar).

**Homocysteine.** A toxic by-product of normal metabolism of an amino acid. High blood levels are associated with vascular disease.

**Hormone.** Various substances formed in endocrine organs which activate specifically receptive organs. Examples are thyroid secretions and insulin.

**Hypoglycemic.** Low blood sugar vs. hyper, high blood sugar.

**Insulin.** Hormone of the pancreas which reduces blood sugar (glucose) and stores this as fat. It also prevents the stored fat from being released.

**Ketosis.** Excessive formation of ketones (organic chemicals) that must be lost through urination. An abnormal fat metabolism occurring in high protein, low carbohydrate diets. This is a controversial diet procedure (the Atkins "Diet Revolution") that many diet professionals malign. It is guarded against in the Zone Diet. It would be a tough diet for lifetime use.

**LBM.** Lean Body Mass

**Lipids.** Fats, such as butter, salad oils, margarine, fat in meat.

**Macronutrient.** The three major nutrients: carbohydrates, proteins, and lipids (fats).

**Mesomorph.** Broad, stocky, muscular physical type.

**Micronutrient.** The minor necessary food components: vitamins and minerals (fibers and water are sometimes labeled "nutrients").

**Monounsaturated fat.** Chemically an "in between" fat that may have advantages over polyunsaturated fats. Both are needed. See Cooper Clinic Tip Sheet for examples. Use olive oil preferentially.

**Orthomolecular Medicine.** Preserving good health and treating disease by varying the concentration in the human body of substances normally present and required for health.

**P/S ratio.** Polyunsaturated fat to saturated fat ratio. A higher value is better. General aim is to strive for a ratio of 1.0. The usual American diet is 0.44.

**Polyunsaturated fat.** Fats that provide the seven unsaturated fatty acids required for life and needed daily. They have "open" carbon atoms that provide life interaction.

**Prostaglandin.** Hormone-like substances derived from fatty acids and found in various body tissues. May affect blood pressure, metabolism, and smooth muscle activity. An eicosanoid.

**Saturated fat.** "Open" carbon atoms "filled" with hydrogen. Many margarines are hydrogenated. They provide nothing but calories.

**Thermogenesis.** Production of animal heat.

**Triglyceride.** Blood fat.

**Zone.** The balance of carbohydrate to protein that stimulates the use of body fat for energy. (See *Glucose*.) Also the feeling that results from this balance because of an even level of blood sugar.

# BIBLIOGRAPHY

Adkins, R. (1972). *Diet Revolution*. David McKay Co.
Applegate, L. (1996). Protein Primer. *Runner's World*. November.
Barnett, R. (1995). The Starch Reality. *The Men's Journal*. Sept.
Batmanghelidj, F. (1995). *Your Body's Many Cries for Water*. Global Health Solutions 800/759-3999.
Bello, F. (1959). How Good Is Mr. Hurley's Diet. *Fortune Magazine*. December.
Blair, et al. (1989). Physical Firtness and All Cause Mortality. *Journal of the American Medical Association*. November 3.
Brant, J. (1987) And the Word Was Aerobics. *Runner's World*
Chait, A. et al. (1993). Rationale of the Diet-Health Statement of the AHA. *American Heart Association Scientific Statement*. Vol. 88, No. 6.
Cimons, M. (1997). Fen-Phen Drug Taken Off Market. *Milwaukee Journal-Sentinel*.
Clouatre, D. & Rosenbaum, M. (1994). *The Diet and Health Benefits of HCA*. New Canaan, CT: Keats Publishing.
Clouatre, D. (1996). *Getting Lean with Anti-fat Nutrients*. San Francisco: Pax Publishing.
*Consumer Reports*. (1992). Eating Right. October.
Cooper, K. (1968). How to Feel Fit at Any Age. *Readers Digest*. March
Cooper, K. (1968). *Aerobics*. New York: M. Evans & Co.
Cooper K. (1970). *The New Aerobics*. New York: M. Evans & Co.
Cooper, K. (1982). *The Aerobics Program for Total Well-Being*. New York: M. Evans & Co.
Cooper, K. (1996). *Advanced Nutritional Therapies*. Nashville, TN: Thomas Nelson, Inc.

Crawford, M. & Marsh, D. (1989). *The Driving Force, Food, Evolution, and the Future.* New York: HarperCollins.

Davis, A. (1954). *Let's Eat Right to Keep Fit.* New York: Harcourt-Brace & Co.

D'Adamo, P.J. with Whitney, C. (1996). *Eat Right for (4) Your Type.* New York: C.P. Putnam's Sons.

Eaton, S.B. & Konner, M. (1985). Paleolithic Nutrition: A Consideration of Its Nature and Current Implications. *New England Journal of Medicine, 312.*

Eaton, S.B., Shostak, M. & Konner, M. (1988). *The Paleolithic Prescription.* New York: HarperCollins.

Friend, T. (1996). Low-fat Diet Isn't Best for Some Men. *USA Today,* July 16.

Gaesser, G. (1996). *Big Fat Lies.* New York: Fawcett Columbine.

Gambaccini, P. (1997). Dumping the Diet. *Runner's World.* January

Gittleman, A. (1996). *Get the Sugar Out.* New York: Crown Publishers, Inc.

Gordon, E. (June, 1969). Obesity: Gluttony or Genes. *Postgraduate Medicine.*

*Harvard Health Letter.* (January 1997).

Katahn, M. (1989). *T-Factor Diet.* New York: W.W. Norton & Co.

Keegan, P. (1997). Dr. Feelbetter. *Outside Magazine,* September.

Kostas, G. G. (1993). *The Balancing Act, Nutrition and Weight Guide.* Kingsport, TN: Quebecor Printing Book Group. (972) 639-7223.

Kostas, G., Miller, K., Kirk, P., Rojohn, K. & Kleckner, C. (1984, 1997). Optimal Nutrition. Cooper Clinic Nutrition Program. Dallas, TX.

Krause, R. et al. (1996). Dietary Guidelines for Healthy American Adults. *American Heart Association Scientific Statement.* Vol. 94, No. 7.

Mackarness, R. (1953). *Eat Fat and Grow Slim.* Garden City, NJ: Doubleday.

McCully, K. (1997). *Homocysteine Revolution.* New Canaan, CN: Keats Publishing, Inc.

Montignac, M. (1991). *Dine Out and Lose Weight.* Montignac USA, Inc., 1531 Colorado Avenue, Santa Monica, CA 90404. To order please call 800/932-3229.

Netzer, C. (1997). *The Complete Book of Food Counts.* New York: Dell Publishing.

Pauling, L. (1970). *Vitamin C and the Common Cold and the Flu.* San Francisco: W.H. Freeman & Co.
Pauling, L. (1986). *How to Live Longer and Feel Better.* New York: W.H. Freeman & Co.
Sears, B. & Lawren, W. (1995). *The Zone, A Dietary Road Map.* New York: Regan Books.
Sears, B. (1997). *Mastering the Zone.* New York: Regan Books.
Sears, B. (1997). *Zone Perfect Meals in Minutes.* New York: Regan Books.
Selye, H. (Rev. 1976). *The Stress of Life.* New York: McGraw-Hill Book Co.
Sevrens, J. (1996). Appetite Suppressant. *Milwaukee Journal Sentinel.* July 8.
Shapiro, L. (1997). Does It Mattter What You Weigh. *Newseek.* April 21.
Sheehan, G. (1975) From the Moment You Become a Spectator Everything is Downhill. *Runners World.*
Sheehan, G. (1980) Medical Advice. *Runners World.* November.
Sheehan, G. (1982) Medical Advice. *Runners World.*
Sheehan, G. (1983) Medical Advice. *Runners World.* August.
Sheehan, G. (1989). *Personal Best.* Emmaus, PA: Rodale Press.
Shils, Olson, & Shike. (1994). *Modern Nutrition in Health and Disease.* 8th edition. Baltimore, MD: Williams & Williams.
Sokolov, R. (1994). Pyramid Power. *Natural History.* January.
*Tufts University Diet and Health Letter.* (May, 1996).
Walford, R. (1986). *The 120-Year Diet.* New York: Simon & Schuster.
Whitaker. J. *The Health and Healing Monthly Report.* Phillips Publishing, 7811 Montrose Road. Potomac, MD 20854. (800) 777-5005.
Wilkholm, G. (1995). From Aerobics to Antioxidants. *Journal of Longevity Research.*

# INDEX

Note: Page numbers followed by "*tbl*" indicate tables, and page numbers followed by "*grph*" indicate graphs.

**Numbers**
*The 120-Year Diet* (Walford), 21–22, 58

**A**
Absorb-A11 Super Formula fat blocker, 68
addictions: Zone diet on, 57
addictive effects of exercise, 92
aerobics, 87–90, 114
   benefits, 90
   point values, 95
   as a stress diversion, 89
agricultural age diet, 3, 121
   diseases from, 2, 120
   and genetic constitution, 1, 2, 3–4
   vs. the Paleolithic diet, 34–48, 117–118
   *See also* Katahn Low Fat diet; modern (American) diet
AHA. *See* American Heart Association
alcohol, 47, 127, 129
   Zone diet on, 57
allergies: from dehydration, 73–75
American diet. *See* modern (American) diet
American Heart Association (AHA)
   on diet, 109
   on sugar, 46

anti-obesity drugs, 67–68
antioxidants, 79
appestat (set point), 14
appetite. *See* hunger
Applegate, Elizabeth: on the RDA of protein, 35–36
arterial disease: Zone diet on, 57
arthritis
   from dehydration, 73
   Zone diet on, 58
asthma: from dehydration, 73–74
autoimmune diseases: Zone diet on, 58

**B**
bad carbohydrates, 19–21, 28*tbl*
bad cholesterol, 42–43
balance in diets, 44
*The Balancing Act, Nutrition and Weight Guide* (Kostas), 63
   fat–cholesterol list, 123–124
Barnett, Bob: "The Starch Reality", 21
Batmanghelidj, Fereydoon
   on dehydration, 72, 84
   on drinking water, 74
beverages, 47, 127
   alcohol, 47, 57, 127, 129
   caffeine, 47, 57, 127, 129
   dehydrating beverages, 74
   soft drinks, 37
   *See also* water
*Big Fat Lies* (Gaesser), 93–94

biochemical measurements of stress, 83
Blair, Steven: on obesity and physical fitness, 93
blood fat levels: and sugars, 70–71
blood sugar levels
    carbohydrate consumption and, 12, 21–22, 27*tbl*, 28*tbl*
    cholesterol levels and, 41–42, 70–71
    and dieting success, 65
    high glycemic foods and, 27
    hyperinsulinism and obesity, 23–26, 29
    hypoglycemia, 20
    weight reduction and, 25*grph*
    Zone diet and, 50–51
blood type diet (D'Adamo), 112
body
    composition, 7
    glycogen stores, 13–14
    metabolic processes and body weight, 13
    physical characteristics of hunter-gatherers, 4
    stature, 3
    types: and dietary needs, 116–117, 118
    *See also* body fat
body fat
    cell size: and insulin levels, 24
    percentages for men and women, 7
    U.S. statistics, 115
    *See also* body fat loss
body fat loss, 64–65
    from exercise, 7, 91
    *See also* weight loss
body types: and dietary needs, 116–117, 118

## C
caffeine, 47, 127, 129
    Zone diet on, 57
calcium, 45, 130
    in the modern and Paleolithic diets, 6

caloric density of foods, 45
calories, 128
    in the Paleolithic diet, 9
    in weight loss plans, 133
    in the Zone diet, 62
cancer prevention
    vitamin C, 78–79
    Zone diet, 58
carbohydrate consumption
    and blood sugar levels, 12, 21–22, 27*tbl*, 28*tbl*
    in the modern and Paleolithic diets, 5, 9
    protein-to-carbohydrate ratio, 56
    and weight gain, 51–53, 70, 80
    in weight loss diets, 14
    Zone diet proportions, 98–99, 125*tbl*
carbohydrates, 9
    bad carbohydrates, 19–21, 28*tbl*
    complex carbohydrates, 21–22, 128
    food counts, 100*tbl*, 101*tbl*
    foods classified as, 29*tbl*
    glycemic index for various types, 27*tbl*, 32–33, 52, 63
    glycogen stores, 13–14
    good carbohydrates, 27–28, 28*tbl*
    grain as a dietary staple, 3, 37, 51
    metabolism of, 21–22, 24
    preferred carbohydrates, 126
    rules for eating, 19–21
    *See also* carbohydrate consumption; sugars
cardiovascular disease
    high blood pressure, 57, 73
    homocysteine levels as indicators, 43–44
    and sugar, 46
    Zone diet on, 57
    *See also* heart disease
chemical food processing: and glycemic index values, 27
cholesterol, 39–44, 114, 127, 128–129

cholesterol *(continued)*
  food counts, 123–124*tbl*
  good and bad types, 42–43
  in the modern and Paleolithic diets, 5, 40
  *See also* cholesterol levels
cholesterol levels, 40, 118
  blood sugar levels and, 41–42, 70–71
  and heart disease, 40–42
  insulin response and, 58
  low cholesterol diets and, 43–44
  low fat diets and, 41
  in males: French vs. U.S., 40
  margarine and, 46
  meat-only diets and, 23
  reducing, 40–44, 67
  weight reduction and, 25–26
  Zone diet and, 61–62
  *See also* cholesterol
Clouatre, Dallas
  on carbohydrates, 53, 70
  on cholesterol levels, 42
  dietary principles, 68–71
  on exercise for weight loss, 70
Clouatre and Rosenbaum: on HCA, 66–67
colitis, 73
complex carbohydrates, 21–22, 128
constipation, 73
*Consumer Reports*: Pyramid diet article, 8*tbl*, 15–16
Cooper, Kenneth
  antioxidant recommendations, 79
  on discipline, 97
  exercise research, 87–90, 92
  water intake recommendations, 75*tbl*
Cooper Clinic
  menu example, 134
  nutrient guide, 128–132
  nutritional guideline tip sheet, 125–127
  Real Life diet, 8*tbl*, 55*tbl*
  weight control guidelines, 133
coronary heart disease. *See* heart disease

## D

D'Adamo, Peter
  on diet for blood type, 112
dairy products, 46
  fats in, 39*tbl*
Davis, Adelle, 115
  on carbohydrates, 22
  nutrition theories, 11, 60–61
death from heart disease: by country, 26*grph*
dehydration
  and disease, 72–74
  stress caused by, 84
desserts, 103
diabetes
  glucose oxidation, 29
  weight reduction and, 25*grph*
  Zone diet on, 57
diet
  balance in, 44
  as evolutionary, 1–10
  and longevity, 58–59
  moderation in, 121
  and stature, 3
  trends in, 11–12
  *See also* dietary guidelines; diets
diet drugs and supplements, 66–68
diet stresses, 83–84
dietary guidelines
  of Adelle Davis, 11, 60–61
  Cooper Clinic nutrient guide, 128–132
  Cooper Clinic tip sheet, 63–64, 125–127
  maintenance diet, 34–48
dietary theories: trends in, 11–12
diets
  Clouatre diet, 68–71
  Cooper Clinic Real Life diet, 8*tbl*
  Hurley diet, 16–17, 115
  Katahn Low Fat diet, 12–15, 99
  maintenance diets, 34–48, 107–108, 119

diets *(continued)*
  McCully diet, 43–44
  meat-only diets, 22–23
  Montignac Low Glycemic diet, 19–21
  Pritikin diet, 44
  USDA diets, 15
  *See also* agricultural age diet; dietary guidelines; Heinrich diet; low fat diets; low glycemic diets; modern (American) diet; Paleolithic diet; Pyramid diet; weight loss diets; Zone diet
digestion. *See* metabolism
digestive system, 1
*Dine Out and Lose Weight* (Montignac), 19
discipline: as an element of success, 97
diseases
  of civilization, 2, 120
  dehydration and, 72–74
  medical treatment for, 122
  from stress, 85–86
  Zone diet on, 57–58, 62–63, 109–112
  *See also* cardiovascular disease; heart disease; preventive health care
diversion of stress, 84–85
drinks. *See* beverages
drugs for weight loss, 66–68
dyspeptic pain, 73

**E**
eating out, 102, 105–106, 118–119
ectomorphs in the weight loss world, 116–117
eicosanoids, 50, 60, 117
  and disease, 57–58
  and fat metabolism, 53, 117
  and protein-to-carbohydrate ratios, 56*grph*
  stress and eicosanoid production, 83–84
elderly people: and exercise, 92

energy level
  exercise and, 92
  HCA and, 67
  Zone diet and, 65, 104–105, 121
evolutionary diet, 1–10
exercise, 91–96, 119–120
  addictive effects, 92
  aerobics, 87–90, 95, 114
  benefits, 90, 92, 98
  and body composition, 7
  and the elderly, 92
  and heart disease, 88–89, 116
  information sources, 96
  and longevity, 88–89, 92–93
  recommended amounts, 89
  repeated, 88
  as a stress equalizer, 84–86, 89
  thermic effects, 13
  walking, 95
  for weight loss, 70, 91–96, 119–120
exercise bicycles, 95

**F**
fast foods, 101*tbl*, 105–106
fat cell size: and insulin levels, 24
fat consumption, 126–127
  and bad carbohydrates, 19
  and cholesterol: in the modern and Paleolithic diets, 5
  dietary recommendations, 54*tbl*
  and hunger, 14
  and insulin levels, 59
  from meats, 36
  in the modern and Paleolithic diets, 5, 9
  and weight gain, 51, 59, 61
  and weight loss, 13–14, 61
  Zone diet proportions, 98–99, 102–103, 125*tbl*
  *See also* fats; low fat diets
fat loss. *See* body fat loss; weight loss
fat–cholesterol list, 123–124*tbl*
fats, 38–39, 128
  burning by exercising, 94–95

fats *(continued)*
  food counts, 100*tbl*, 101*tbl*, 123–124*tbl*
  foods classified as, 29*tbl*
  margarine, 46
  from meat and dairy products, 39*tbl*
  metabolism of, 53, 94
  nutritional value, 52
  saturated/unsaturated fats, 38–39
  *See also* body fat; fat consumption
fiber, 45, 126, 129
  foods classified as, 29*tbl*
  in the modern and Paleolithic diets, 5
fitness. *See* physical fitness
folic acid, 44, 132
food counts, 47, 99–103, 100*tbl*
  fast foods, 101*tbl*
  fats, 100*tbl*, 101*tbl*, 123–124*tbl*
food processing: and glycemic index values, 27
foods
  beverages, 37, 47
  dairy products, 39*tbl*, 46
  as drugs, 59–60, 68
  fast foods, 101*tbl*, 105–106
  fiber, 45, 126
  grain, 3, 37, 51
  as macronutrients, 29*tbl*, 50
  meat, 35–36
  minerals, 45, 130–131
  Montignac diet food classifications, 30*tbl*, 31*tbl*
  nutrient guide, 128–132
  plant foods, 36–37
  processed foods, 27, 46–47
  salt, 45, 127, 130
  shopping for, 47
  thermic effects, 13
  wild foods, 4
  *See also* carbohydrates; cholesterol; diet; diets; fats; food counts; nutrition guidelines; protein; sugars; vitamins; water

four food groups (USDA diets), 15
Friend, Tim: on low fat diets for men, 41
fructose, 37–38
  and cholesterol levels, 70–71
  and heart disease, 41–42
fruits, 36–37

# G
Gaesser, Glenn: *Big Fat Lies*, 93–94
gaining weight. *See* weight gain
GAS (General Adaptation System), 83
General Adaptation System (GAS), 83
genetic constitution
  and the agricultural age diet, 1, 2, 3–4
  and the glycemic index, 33
  and health, 94
  insulin response, 51–52
  and weight loss, 10
*Getting Lean with Anti-Fat Nutrients* (Clouatre), 68–71
Gittelman, A.: on grocery shopping, 47
glucagon, 50
glucose
  metabolism of, 23, 36, 37–38
  nutritional value, 52
  oxidation in diabetics, 29
glycemic index, 15, 20–23, 32–33
  of carbohydrates, 27*tbl*, 32–33, 52, 63
  chemical food processing and, 27
  and heart disease, 25–26, 26*grph*
  physiology, 32
  and the Pyramid diet, 119
  scientific acceptance of, 113
  *See also* low glycemic diets
glycogen stores, 13–14
  increasing, 67
good carbohydrates, 27–28, 28*tbl*
good cholesterol, 42–43

Gordon, Edgar
  on fats, 52
  on obesity, 23–24, 29
grain: as a dietary staple, 3, 37, 51
grocery shopping, 47

## H

HCA (hydroxycitric acid), 66–67
*Health & Healing* monthly report, 96
health care: medical treatment for diseases, 122
  *See also* preventive health care
heart disease
  cholesterol levels and, 40–42
  death from: by country, 26*grph*
  from diet drugs, 68
  exercise and, 88–89, 116
  homocysteine levels as indicators, 43–44
  hypoglycemic foods and, 25–26, 26*grph*
  insulin production and, 33
  LDL and, 79
  risk factors, 93
  sugar consumption and, 41, 46, 78
  vitamin C and, 79–81
  Zone diet and, 109–112
  *See also* cardiovascular disease
heartburn, 73
Heinrich diet, 97–108, 113–114, 121–122
  eating out, 102, 105–106, 118–119
  energy level, 104–105
  menu example, 104
  snacks, 104
  tips, 106–107
high blood pressure
  dehydration and, 73
  Zone diet on, 57
high glycemic foods: and blood sugar levels, 27
homocysteine levels, 43–44

*Homocysteine Revolution* (McCully), 43–44
hormones from food, 59–60
hunger
  controlling, 14, 67, 73
  fat consumption and, 14
hunter-gatherers
  eating patterns, 7
  physical characteristics, 4
Hurley diet, 16–17, 115
hydroxycitric acid (HCA), 66–67
hyperinsulinism: obesity and, 23–24
hypertension. *See* high blood pressure
hypoglycemia: obesity and, 20
hypoglycemic foods: and heart disease, 25–26, 26*grph*

## I

insulin, 50
insulin levels
  diet and, 110
  fat consumption and, 59
  and heart disease, 33
  maintaining safe levels, 110
  obesity and, 23–26
  and the Pyramid diet, 119
  weight loss and, 25*grph*
  *See also* glycemic index; insulin response
insulin response, 51–52
  and cholesterol levels, 58
iron, 131

## K

Katahn, Martin: on what makes you fat, 51
Katahn Low Fat diet, 12–15, 40
  metabolic factors, 13–15
  parameters, 12–13
  Zone diet vs., 99
Keegan, Paul: on the Zone diet, 64, 65
ketosis: from meat-only diets, 22–23
Keys, Ancel: weight loss study, 91

Kostas, Georgia G.
*The Balancing Act, Nutrition and Weight Guide*, 63
fat–cholesterol list, 123–124*tbl*
nutrient guide, 128–132
nutrition tip sheet, 63–64, 125–127

**L**
LAS (Local Adaptation Syndrome), 83
LDL (low density lipoproteins), 43
and heart disease, 79
*Let's Eat Right to Keep Fit* (Davis), 60–61
lipogenesis inhibition from HCA, 67
Local Adaptation Syndrome (LAS), 83
longevity
diet and, 58–59
exercise and, 88–89, 92–93
losing weight. *See* weight loss; weight loss diets
low cholesterol diets: McCully diet, 43–44
low density lipoproteins. *See* LDL
low fat diets, 11–17
and cholesterol levels, 41
Katahn Low Fat diet, 12–15
for men, 40–42
usefulness for various metabolic types, 14–15
Zone diet as, 56
low glycemic diets, 18–33
bad carbohydrates, 19–21, 28*tbl*
glycemic index, 15, 20–23, 25–27, 27*grph*, 32–33
good carbohydrates, 27–28, 28*tbl*
McCully diet, 43–44
Montignac Low Glycemic diet, 19–21
social eating and, 102
*See also* Zone diet

**M**
macronutrients
foods classified as, 29*tbl*
proper mix, 50
*See also* carbohydrates; fats; food counts; protein
magnesium, 130
maintenance diets, 34–48, 107–108, 119
margarine, 46
McCully diet, 43–44
meat, 35–36
fats in, 39*tbl*
meat-only diets, 22–23
medical treatment for diseases, 122
men
cholesterol levels: French vs. American, 40
low fat diets for, 40–42
menu examples for weight loss diets, 69–71, 104, 134
metabolism
of carbohydrates, 21–22
of fats, 53, 117
of glucose, 23, 36, 37–38
obesity as a metabolic defect, 23–26, 29
weight loss factors, 13–15, 20–23
methioinine: minimizing, 44
minerals, 45, 130–131
moderation in diet, 121
modern (American) diet, 7–8
calcium intake, 6
carbohydrate consumption, 5, 9
cholesterol intake, 5
diseases from, 2, 120
fat consumption, 5, 9
fiber intake, 5
four food groups, 15
male cholesterol levels, 40
P/S Ratio, 5
vs. the Paleolithic diet, 4–10, 6*tbl*, 8*tbl*
potassium intake, 6
problems of, 7–8

modern (American) diet *(cont.)*
    protein consumption, 5, 9
    vitamin C intake, 6
    *See also* agricultural age diet; Pyramid Diet, USDA
*Modern Nutrition in Health and Disease* (Shils, Olson, and Shike), 32
mono-unsaturated fats, 39, 126–127
Montignac Low Glycemic diet, 12, 19–21, 40, 118–119
    allowed food classifications, 30*tbl*, 31*tbl*
    vs. other diets, 69–71
    *See also* glycemic index
muscularity: as a health factor, 7

## N

National Cancer Institute (NCI): vitamin C research, 78–79
NCI. *See* National Cancer Institute
Neo-Paleolithic diets. *See* Paleolithic diet
Netzer food counts, 47, 100*tbl*, 101*tbl*
niacin (vitamin $B_3$), 132
nutrient density, 45
nutrient guide: Cooper Clinic, 128–132
    *See also* dietary guidelines
nutrition. *See* diet; foods

## O

obesity
    anti-obesity drugs, 67–68
    dehydration and, 73
    and hyperinsulinism, 23–24
    and hypoglycemia, 20
    as a metabolic defect, 23–26, 29
    and physical fitness, 93
    Zone diet on, 57
*The 120-Year Diet* (Walford), 21–22, 58
overeating: as a survival mechanism, 7

## P

P/S Ratio: in the modern and Paleolithic diets, 5
Paleolithic diet, 1–10, 114–115, 121–122
    vs. the agricultural age diet, 34–48, 117–118
    calcium intake, 6
    caloric content, 9
    carbohydrate consumption, 5, 9
    cholesterol intake, 5
    vs. the Clouatre diet, 68–71
    fat consumption, 5, 9
    fiber intake, 5
    vs. the modern (American) diet, 4–10, 6*tbl*, 8*tbl*
    P/S Ratio, 5
    potassium intake, 6
    protein consumption, 5, 9
    vitamin C intake, 6
pantothenic acid, 132
Pauling, Linus, 76, 81
    on carbohydrates, 53, 80
    diet and fitness recommendations, 107–108
    on sugar, 37
    vitamin C research, 77–79
    on vitamins, 78, 81
    on water, 74
phosphorus, 130
physical fitness
    from exercise, 88–96
    and longevity, 93
    and obesity, 93
    for various body types, 116–117
    *See also* exercise
plant foods, 36–37
polyunsaturated fats, 38–39, 126
    P/S Ratio in the modern and Paleolithic diets, 5
Pondimin anti-obesity drug, 68
potassium, 130
    in the modern and Paleolithic diets, 6
prepared foods. *See* fast foods; processed (prepared) foods

preventive health care
  exercise as, 87–90
  information sources, 96
  water drinking as, 72–74
  Zone diet as, 57–58, 62–63, 109–112
  *See also* diseases
Pritikin diet: criticisms of, 44
processed (prepared) foods, 27, 46–47
  *See also* fast foods
prostaglandin, 57
protein, 52–53, 128
  food counts, 100*tbl*, 101*tbl*
  foods classified as, 29*tbl*
  *See also* protein consumption
protein consumption
  and homocysteine levels, 43
  in the modern and Paleolithic diets, 5, 9
  protein-to-carbohydrate ratio, 56
  recommended amounts, 35–36, 54*tbl*, 114
  Zone diet proportions, 98–99, 125*tbl*
  *See also* protein
protein-to-carbohydrate ratio, 56
Pyramid diet, USDA, 15–16, 116
  as a weight loss diet, 119
  Zone diet vs., 63–64, 99
pyridoxine (vitamin B$_6$), 44, 132

**R**
RDA (Recommended Daily Allowance): of protein, 35–36
Recommended Daily Allowance (RDA) of protein, 35–36
reducing diets. *See* weight loss diets
Redux anti-obesity drug, 67–68
requirements for various foods. *See* RDA; *and specific foods and macronutrients*
restaurant meals, 102, 105–106
rheumatoid arthritis: from dehydration, 73
riboflavin (vitamin B$_2$), 131

**S**
salt, 45, 127, 130
saturated fats, 38, 113–114
  P/S Ratio in the modern and Paleolithic diets, 5
scientific community: acceptance of health research, 113–115
Sears, Barry, 57
  on carbohydrates, 51, 52, 94
  on cholesterol, 42–43, 46, 58
  on eicosanoids, 50, 60
  on exercise, 95
  on food, 59–60, 68
  on the Paleolithic diet, 118
  on stress, 83–84
  on U.S. eating habits, 59–60
  on what makes you fat, 51
  on the Zone diet, 49–50, 94
Sears Zone Reducing diet. *See* Zone diet
Selye, Hans
  on stress, 85
  stress research, 82–83
Senate-recommended diet, 8*tbl*
serum cholesterol levels. *See* cholesterol levels
set point (appestat), 14
Shapiro, Laura: on obesity and physical fitness, 93
Sheehan, George
  on stress and stress diversion, 86
  on weight loss, 91
Shils, Olson, and Shike: on the glycemic index, 32
shopping for foods, 47
simple carbohydrates. *See* sugars
skipping meals, 14
sleep: stress and, 85
smoking: Zone diet on, 57
snacking, 104
social eating, 102, 105–106
sodium, 45, 127, 130
soft drinks, 37
spectator sports: stressful aspects, 86
spinal pain: from dehydration, 73

starch. *See* carbohydrates
"The Starch Reality" (Barnett), 21
stature: nutrition and, 3
stress, 82–86
   biochemical measurements of, 83
   diversion of, 84–85, 89
   illness from, 85–86
   mechanics, 83–84
   relieving, 127
   scientific acceptance of, 113
   signs, 85
   and sleep, 85
*The Stress of Life* (Selye), 82
sugars, 37–38, 127, 129
   and blood fat levels, 70–71
   consumption through history, 78
   and heart disease, 41–42, 46, 78
   U.S. consumption, 37–38
supplements for weight loss, 66–68

## T

T-Factor Diet. *See* Katahn Low Fat Diet
thermic effects of foods and exercise, 13
thermogenesis, 13
   HCA and, 67
thiamin (vitamin $B_1$), 131
trace minerals, 45, 130
training table, maintenance diet, 34–48

## U

United States
   body fat statistics, 115
   male cholesterol levels, 40
   sugar consumption statistics, 37–38
   *See also* modern (American) diet
unsaturated fats, 38–39
USDA diets: four food groups, 15
   *See also* Pyramid diet, USDA

## V

vegetables, 36–37
vitamin A, 131
vitamin $B_1$ (thiamin), 131
vitamin $B_2$ (riboflavin), 131
vitamin $B_3$ (niacin), 132
vitamin $B_6$ (pyridoxine), 44, 132
vitamin $B_{12}$, 44, 132
vitamin C, 45, 77–79, 114
   actions of, 77, 132
   and cancer, 78–79
   and heart disease, 79–81
   in the modern and Paleolithic diets, 6
   Pauling's theories, 77–79
   recommended intake, 79, 81
   safety, 77
   sources, 81, 132
*Vitamin C and the Common Cold and the Flu* (Pauling), 77–78
vitamin D, 131
vitamin E, 44, 131
vitamins, 44, 78, 114, 131–132
   sources for, 81
   *See also* vitamin C

## W

Walford, Roy: *The 120-Year Diet*, 21–22, 58
walking, 95
water, 72–75, 114, 120, 129
   daily requirements, 74–75, 75*tbl*, 129
   diseases prevented and treated by, 72–74, 120
   stress caused by, 84
water retention: from dehydration, 73
weight control guidelines: Cooper Clinic, 133
weight gain
   from carbohydrates, 51–53, 70
   from fats, 51, 59, 61
   *See also* weight loss
weight loss
   and blood sugar levels, 25*grph*, 65
   body fat loss, 64–65
   and cholesterol levels, 25–26

# INDEX

weight loss *(continued)*
  from drinking water, 73
  drugs for, 66–68
  exercise as a key to, 70, 91–96, 119–120
  fat consumption and, 13–14, 61
  guidelines, 133
  and insulin levels, 25*grph*
  metabolic factors, 13, 20–23, 23–26
  supplements for, 66–68
  Zone diet and, 64–65
  *See also* weight loss diets
weight loss diets, 11–17
  body type and dietary needs, 116–117, 118
  Clouatre diet, 68–71
  comparisons, 8*tbl*, 54–57, 54*tbl*, 55*tbl*, 63–64, 69–71, 99–103
  desserts, 103
  diabetic blood levels affected by, 25*grph*
  eating out, 102, 105–106, 118–119
  and fat consumption, 13–14, 54*tbl*
  fat recommendations, 54*tbl*
  food counts, 47, 99–103, 100*tbl*, 101*tbl*
  and genetic constitution, 10
  glycemic index, 15
  Heinrich diet, 97–108, 113–114, 121–122
  Hurley diet, 16–17, 115
  Katahn Low Fat diet, 12–15
  low fat diets, 11–17
  low glycemic diets, 18–33
  maintenance diets, 34–48, 107–108, 119
  meat-only diets, 22–23
  menu examples, 69–71, 104, 134
  Montignac Low Glycemic diet, 19–21
  protein recommendations, 54*tbl*
  Pyramid diet as, 15–16, 63–64, 99, 119
  skipping meals, 14
  snacks, 104
  tips, 106–107
  *See also* exercise; hunger; weight loss; Zone diet
weight maintenance: allowed foods, 31*tbl*
Whitaker, Julian: *The Health and Healing* monthly report, 96
wild foods: as natural, 4

**Z**

zinc, 130–131
Zone, 50–51
  stress and, 83–84
Zone diet, 49–65
  benefits, 50, 55, 59–63, 65, 98, 104–105, 109–112, 121
  and blood sugar levels, 50–51
  caloric content, 62
  carbohydrate stance, 51–53
  and cholesterol levels, 61–62
  criticisms of, 54, 61–63, 64
  eating out, 105–106
  epidemiological studies, 111–112
  individualized diets, 53–54, 56–57, 63–64, 104, 105, 106–107
  menu examples, 104
  vs. other diets, 8*tbl*, 54–57, 54*tbl*, 55*tbl*, 63–64, 99–103
  precepts, 103
  as a preventive health measure, 57–58, 62–63, 109–112
  protein-to-carbohydrate ratios, 55*tbl*, 56*grph*
  studies needed, 110–112
  and weight loss, 64–65
  wellness conclusions, 59–60

## RICHARD L. HEINRICH,

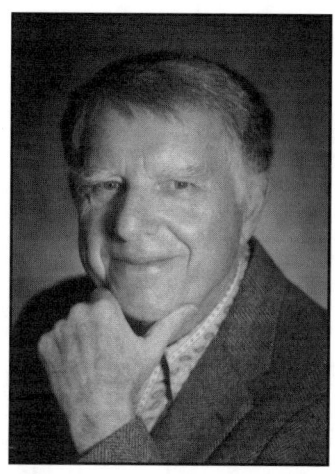

at 72, knows science and the scientific approach. He was an ensign at age 20 and a teacher of thermodynamics at 21, while earning his M.S. in Mechanical Engineering from the University of Wisconsin.

After stints at Douglas Aircraft (even a junior assignment on the X-2) and as a project engineer at Oscar Mayer, he commenced businesses in sales, engineering, and manufacturing bridge cranes.

He struggled with a life-long weight problem, investigating a half century of diet and fitness, and studied the wellness teachings of those who became his personal heroes. This book becomes his legacy. He says, "I can't leave an art museum, but perhaps the knowledge I've acquired in fifty years of questing after fitness and wellness is actually more lasting. It can be expanded upon by others and, when disputed, may lead to a greater set of truths."

He's walked the walk, now he talks the talk!